ATLAS OF
MINOR
SURGERY

For Churchill Livingstone:

Publisher: Timothy Horne
Project Editor: Janice Urquhart
Copy Editor: Jennifer Bew
Project Controller: Kay Hunston
Design Direction: Judith Wright

ATLAS OF
MINOR SURGERY

Ian D. Cracknell MB BS LRCP MRCS
General Practitioner, Hinckley; Hospital Practitioner in General Surgery,
Fosse Health Trust, UK

Michael G. Mead BSc MB BS DCH DRCOG MRCGP
General Practitioner, Leicester, UK

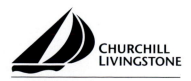

CHURCHILL
LIVINGSTONE

NEW YORK EDINBURGH LONDON MADRID MELBOURNE SAN FRANCISCO AND TOKYO 1997

CHURCHILL LIVINGSTONE
Medical Division of Pearson Professional Limited

Distributed in the United States of America by Churchill
Livingstone Inc., 650 Avenue of the Americas, New York,
N.Y. 10011, and by associated companies, branches and
representatives throughout the world.

First published 1997

ISBN 0 443 05304 9

British Library Cataloguing in Publication Data
A catalogue record for this book is available from the
British Library

Library of Congress Cataloging in Publication Data
A catalog record for this book is available from the
Library of Congress

Medical knowledge is constantly changing. As new
information becomes available, changes in treatment,
procedures, equipment and the use of drugs become
necessary. The authors and the publishers have, as far
as it is possible, taken care to ensure that the
information given in the text is accurate and up to date.
However, readers are strongly advised to confirm that
the information, especially with regard to drug usage,
complies with current legislation and standards of
practice.

The
publisher's
policy is to use
**paper manufactured
from sustainable forests**

Produced by Longman Asia Ltd, Hong Kong

Contents

Preface

Minor surgery is part of the everyday practice of many doctors. Whether injecting a joint, lancing an abscess or removing a skin tag, minor surgery procedures are among the commonest clinical activities. Even budding surgical specialists need to start with removing sebaceous cysts and lipomas, injecting haemorrhoids and aspirating breast cysts.

This book covers all the minor surgery procedures one would expect to be carried out in a community setting, together with a few more advanced procedures (like vasectomy) for those family doctors who wish to extend their surgical skills. It should serve as a practical manual for all those doctors, both established and in training, who intend to offer their patients a minor surgery service. The logical (and cost effective) place for minor surgery is in the treatment room of a family doctor's practice. The expansion of such locally-based services is where the future of medicine lies.

1997   I. D. C.
                                                                                 M. G. M.

Acknowledgements

We would like to thank all our colleagues who have helped in the preparation of this book. Particular thanks go to the two principal photographers, Sasha Andrew and Adrian Jefferies, and to the following consultants who have both provided illustrations and advice: Mr G. Fahy, Consultant Ophthalmologist, Leicester Royal Infirmary; Mr H. Henderson, Consultant Plastic Surgeon, Leicester Royal Infirmary; Mr G. Murty, Consultant ENT Surgeon, Leicester Royal Infirmary; Mr D. Rew and Mr A. Scott, both Consultant Surgeons at Glenfield General Hospital.

We would also like to thank Reed Healthcare Publishing for permission to reproduce illustrations from the series on minor surgery in general practice which appeared in Update in and around 1991.

Finally we would like to thank the European Resuscitation Council for permission to reproduce material on cardiac life support.

1997

I. D. C.
M. G. M.

1 Minor surgery in practice

Procedures

Minor surgery means different procedures to different doctors. Conditions for which minor surgery is appropriate, such as an ingrowing toenail (Fig. 1) or a pigmented naevus (Fig. 2), rank among the commonest of all presentations to a family doctor. Be sure of your diagnosis before operating, however – these common conditions can occasionally be confused with more serious pathology (Fig. 3). The key to success is to attempt only those procedures you feel confident with (and have been properly trained for).

The following procedures, which qualify for an NHS payment under the UK scheme, are a good starting point. Doctors in family practice should aim for a proficiency in these areas before considering whether they wish to train for more difficult surgery.

- Injections: intra-articular, periarticular, injection of varicose veins and haemorrhoids

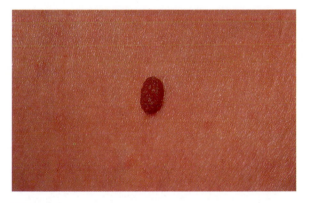

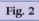

Fig. 2

A simple pigmented naevus: ideal territory for minor surgery.

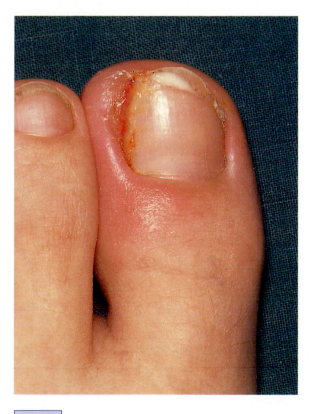

Fig. 1

Ingrowing toenail: one of the commonest conditions requiring minor surgery.

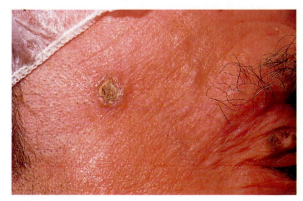

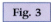

Fig. 3

Squamous cell carcinoma: be sure of your diagnosis before attempting minor surgery.

- Aspirations: joints, cysts, bursae, hydrocoeles
- Incisions: abscesses, cysts, thrombosed piles
- Excisions: sebaceous cysts, intradermal naevi, papilloma, dermatofibroma, warts, skin lesions for histology, lipomas, partial or complete toenail removal
- Cautery/curetting: warts, verrucas, other skin lesions (including cryocautery), nasal cautery
- Removal of foreign bodies.

In the authors' view the treatment of varicose veins in the setting of family practice should be discouraged, and this procedure will not be covered in this book.

Training

Training is essential, ideally by attachment to a local surgeon to gain supervised 'hands-on' experience. Courses containing practical demonstrations of minor surgical techniques are also useful. Once trained, there is also an obligation to maintain and update one's surgical skills. In a partnership of doctors not all will wish to attempt the more complicated procedures such as vasectomy (Fig. 4). The best strategy is to have one doctor in the group trained for procedures demanding higher surgical expertise, and to train one doctor in advanced techniques, such as sigmoidoscopy, rather than

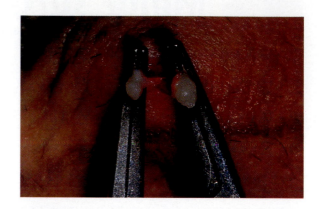

Fig. 4

Tips of the vas deferens: vasectomy is one of the more advanced minor surgery procedures.

have each partner performing the techniques incompetently.

Liaison with local specialists

In whatever context you are undertaking minor surgery it is important to establish a link with your local surgical teams and pathologists. During your career you will be sure to need their advice and support, and it is reassuring to have ready access to a surgical unit in case of unexpected difficulties.

2 Medicolegal issues

Consent

Informed consent is a cornerstone of good practice. The patient should be given a clear explanation of the nature and purpose of the operation, together with anticipated postoperative care and a brief discussion of possible complications. It is sensible for all but the most minor procedures to use a consent form (Fig. 5), which will also serve as a record of the procedure. Special care and attention must be given to ensure informed consent in the case of

---

CONSENT FOR OPERATION

I _____ of _____

_____

Hereby consent to * undergo   * child
                   * submission of my   * ward
the operation of _____
the nature and purpose of which has been explained to me by
Dr _____
I also consent to such further or alternative operative measures as may
be found necessary during the course of the above mentioned operation
and to the administration of local or other anaesthetics for any of
these purposes.
No assurance has been given to me that the operation will be performed
by any particular practitioner.
Date _____   Signed _____
                                       (patient/partner/guardian*)
I confirm that I have explained the nature and purpose of this operation
to the patient/partner/guardian*
Date _____   Signed _____
                                       Medical practitioner

* DELETE AS APPROPRIATE

Any deletions, insertions or amendments to the form are to be made
before the explanation is given and the form submitted for signature.

Fig. 5

A good example of a consent form for minor surgery.

children and the mentally handicapped. If the patient has a limited command of the English language, an interpreter may be required. Similarly, it may be difficult to obtain informed consent from those with a severe psychiatric disorder.

Keeping good records

It is essential to keep good records of the procedure carried out, when it was carried out, which area of the body was operated on, what anaesthetic was used and who was the operating surgeon.

Defence cover

It is also essential to have adequate defence cover from a reliable medical defence organization before embarking on any minor surgery.

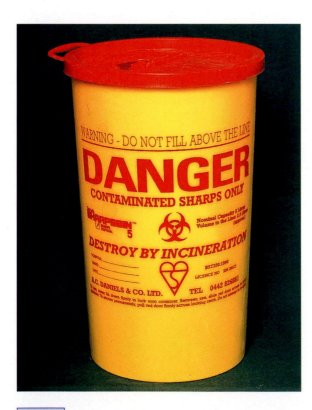

Fig. 6
A sharps container.

Histological diagnosis

Whenever a lump or lesion is excised, it is a wise policy to send the specimen in a preservative (e.g. a 10% formalin pot) to the local pathology laboratory for an accurate histological diagnosis. It is not necessary to send lipomas, sebaceous cysts or toenails for histology.

Prevention of infection

It is important to ensure that infection is not introduced as a result of poor practice standards. Infection can work both ways – the operator acquiring infection as a result of contact with a patient's body fluids, and the patient acquiring infection from non-sterile surgical technique. Prevention of infection means personal cleanliness (including scrubbing up), the use of surgical gloves and adequate sterilization of instruments (see p. 5).

Hepatitis B immunization

Those undertaking minor surgery, including those assisting, should be fully immunized against hepatitis B.

Waste disposal

A practice undertaking minor surgery must also have facilities to dispose of the clinical waste, which may act as a source of infection. Sharps containers (Fig. 6) are essential.

Good practice

Doctors will also wish to be guided by current consensus on good practice. Observe closely the contraindications to anaesthesia.

Patient suitability

The following patient groups may not be deemed suitable for surgery in the family practice setting: diabetics, patients on steroids, those with a psychiatric disorder, those with a bleeding tendency, immunosuppressed patients, those with transmissible infections and children.

Premises and equipment

Treatment room

A spacious area (Fig. 7) must be set aside for minor surgery, free from any potential source of dust or contamination. This need not be a separate room – it may be possible to screen off an area of a treatment room for minor surgery.

The importance of good lighting cannot be overstated. What is required is high-intensity overhead and sidelighting. Wall- or ceiling-mounted theatre lights (as illustrated in Fig. 7) are the best source of lighting for minor surgery.

The couch/operating table should be adjustable and set at a height that gives the surgeon ease of access without undue bending or strain.

Sterilization

Surgery obviously requires sterile surgical equipment and this is best achieved by steam sterilization at 134–138°C at 2. 2 bar gauge steam pressure for 3–$3\frac{1}{2}$ minutes. It may be possible to contract this service from your local hospital, but for the majority of doctors in the community the most appropriate course of action is to purchase a benchtop sterilizer.

The sterilizer (Fig. 8) should be properly installed and will require an insurance certificate, which must be renewed by inspection after a statutory interval. A good maintenance programme is essential, with regular visits from a maintenance engineer.

The nurse responsible for the sterilization procedure must record a daily check of the sterilization cycle, including temperature, steam pressure and time.

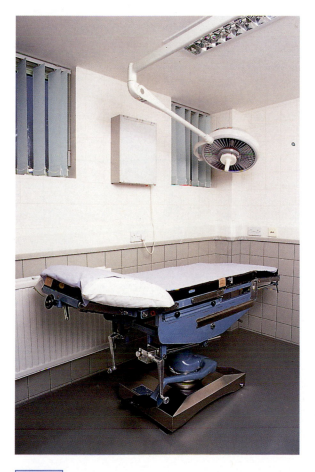

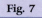
Fig. 7

The ideal situation for minor surgery: a spacious area, adjustable couch and adequate lighting.

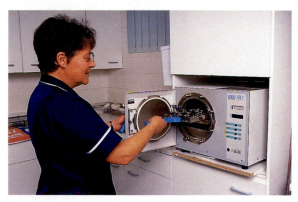

Fig. 8

A sterilizer is essential for any surgical practice.

Cautery/Cryocautery

Hot-wire cautery equipment is useful if used judiciously to control bleeding, and is a worthwhile addition to your equipment portfolio.

Cryocautery is a valuable technique for destroying superficial skin lesions such as verrucae and warts, and cryocautery equipment (Fig. 9) should form part of any minor surgery kit. Cottonwool buds can be used to apply liquid nitrogen to a lesion, but the most satisfactory method is to use a cryoprobe (e.g. by means of the Cryojet, which can also deliver a spray). Although expensive to purchase, the equipment will pay for itself over time with the throughput of patients in your skin lesion clinic.

If you are undertaking cryotherapy to any degree, you will also need a Dewar flask (Fig. 10) to store the liquid nitrogen, otherwise this means a daily/weekly trip to the hospital with a transit flask full of liquid nitrogen.

An alternative for cryocautery is the use of a Histofreezer, a disposable aerosol spray used in conjunction with a bud (i.e. it is similar to employing a cottonwool bud dipped in liquid nitrogen).

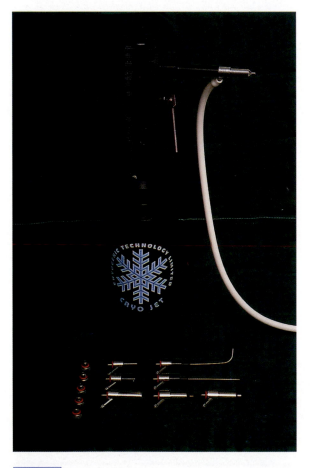

Fig. 9

Cryocautery equipment: a valuable asset for minor surgery.

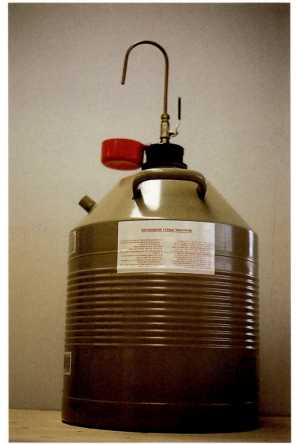

Fig. 10

A Dewar flask for storing liquid nitrogen.

4 Surgical instruments

Every surgeon will have a slightly different selection of instruments, based on personal preference, but the following constitute a minor surgery set:

- Scissors (small, curved dissecting)
- Scissors (large straight)
- Forceps (fine, toothed dissecting)
- Forceps (fine, non-toothed dissecting)
- Scalpel handle (sizes 10, 11 and 15)
- Mosquito forceps (two pairs)
- Large artery forceps (two pairs)

- Gillies suture holders or small smooth-bladed suture holder
- Cat's-paw retractor
- Allis's tissue-holding forceps
- Curettes (large and small)
- Blunt probe
- Skin hooks
- Scalpel blades and sutures
- Skin closure strips.

It is a false economy to purchase cheap instruments – high-quality instruments will give you several years of use and, since minor surgery is largely fine work, will also assist you in achieving better results. Remember not to leave instruments in the sterilizer. Scissors should ideally be hot-air or spirit cleaned rather than autoclaved.

Figures 11–13 show a representative selection of surgical instruments thus: Fig. 11: From left to right: fine suture holders, long curved dissecting scissors, Gillies suture holder, straight heavy scissors, short fine-curved dissecting scissors; Fig. 12: From left to right: fine-toothed dissecting forceps, fine non-toothed dissecting forceps, towel clip, mosquito forceps, tissue-holding forceps, vasectomy forceps; Fig. 13: From left to right: curette, retractors (two), skin hooks (two), scalpel handle.

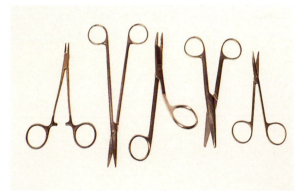

Fig. 11

Surgical instruments (see text for details).

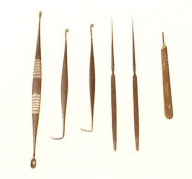

Fig. 12

Surgical instruments (see text for details).

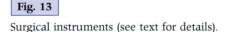

Fig. 13

Surgical instruments (see text for details).

As with instruments, the drapes used for surgery are a matter of personal preference. Drapes are desirable for a sterile operating field but they will not be essential for many of the more minor surgical cases.

Hyfrecation

Hyfrecator equipment is now readily available and offers the best means of controlling minor haemorrhage in the practice environment. The hyfrecator (Fig. 14) has a facility for bipolar coagulation, which is extremely useful for the purposes of treating superficial skin lesions (much in the same way as hot-wire cautery or cryocautery), as well as securing haemostasis during a surgical procedure.

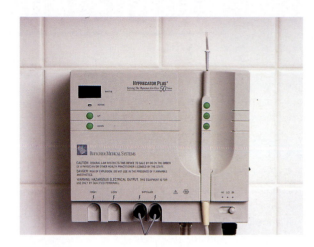

Fig. 14

A hyfrecator.

Surgical blades and sutures

Blades

Three types of surgical blade will suffice: numbers 10, 11 and 15. A small scalpel blade , such as a size 15, should be used for most lesions, incising along a line of cleavage where possible. The incision should be made with the knife held at right-angles to the skin.

Type of blade	Uses
Number 11	Suture removal
	Vasectomy
Number 15	All small lesions
	Biopsy (incisional and excisional)
	Minor cosmetic procedures
Number 10	Ingrowing toenails
	Larger lesions (e.g. lipomas)

Sutures

Four types of suture material should suffice: 4/0 plain catgut, 4/0 Vicryl, 4/0 Ethilon and 6/0 Ethilon. Prolene can be used instead of Ethilon. The wound should be closed with the smallest suture compatible with the site and tension of the wound. For a gaping wound use a subcuticular absorbable 4/0 undyed Vicryl or Dexon stitch to relieve the tension of the surface skin suturing.

Type of suture		Uses
4/0	Plain catgut (absorbable)	Subcutaneous wound approximation
		Fat suture
		Skin closure (e.g. vasectomy)
4/0	Undyed Vicryl or Dexon (absorbable)	Subcutaneous wound closure
		Subcuticular suture
		Ligation of vasa
		Dead-space obliteration (e.g. large lipoma)
4/0	Non-absorbable monofilament	Wound closure (trunk and limbs)
6/0	Non-absorbable monofilament	Wound closure (face and hands).

Figure 15 illustrates the various blades and sutures and Figure 16 shows Prolene sutures in place. Figure 17 shows skin closure strips. When used properly skin closure strips have a wide range of uses. If

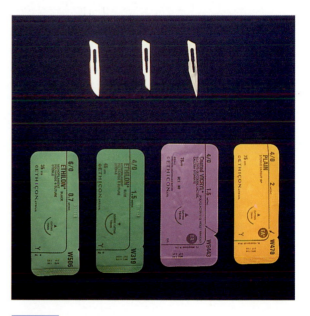

Fig. 15

Blades and sutures.

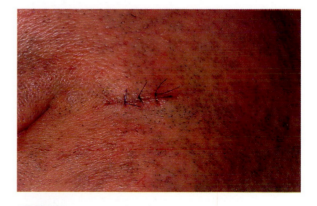

Fig. 16

6/0 Prolene sutures in place.

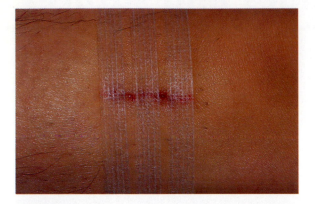

Fig. 17

Skin closure strips.

wound edges are approximated with a subcuticular or subcutaneous stitch, skin closure strips can sometimes be used to avoid using a skin suture, e.g. in a patient susceptible to keloid formation. Skin closure strips are also useful for approximating small lacerations in children – never the easiest patients for fine skin suturing!

6 Local anaesthetics and topical agents

Local anaesthesia

Lignocaine 1% is adequate in most situations. For wide infiltration of a large area use 0.5% lignocaine. The lignocaine should be infiltrated prior to scrubbing up to allow adequate time (at least 5–10 minutes) for it to take effect or, if adrenaline is used, for the ischaemia to occur. Lignocaine plus adrenaline is useful for the scalp and face (not the nose or ears), the adrenaline assisting in achieving a bloodless field. Adrenaline should *never* be used in a ring block or in the extremities (digits, nose, ears, penis).

It is important to learn the correct technique of infiltration with local anaesthetic. There are 10 rules to remember:

1. Always use the finest needle you can – a dental syringe is ideal.
2. Always use the least amount of drug to give satisfactory anaesthesia.
3. Aspirate before infiltration (although this will not be possible if you use a dental syringe).
4. Infiltrate while moving the needle, preferably through a plane of previously anaesthetized tissue.
5. Always infiltrate widely around the lesion to be removed.
6. If at all possible avoid infiltrating directly into a lesion.
7. Remember the safe maximum dose of local anaesthetic is 20 ml of 1% lignocaine.
8. When using adrenaline the degree of blanching will correlate with the extent of anaesthesia.
9. Local anaesthetic agents should preferably be used in the form of individual patient ampoules.
10. Always enter in the medical records the type of anaesthetic used and the batch number.

The enzyme hyaluronidase (Hyalase) may be used with the local anaesthetic in ring blocks, but, as it is derived from eggs, remember to ask the patient about sensitivity to eggs.

A few patients are very sensitive to lignocaine, or else it fails to achieve adequate analgesia. In these situations we would use bupivacaine. This is slower in onset of action than lignocaine but its effects last longer. Bupivacaine is particularly useful for regional blocks.

An ethyl chloride spray is occasionally useful as an anaesthetic agent when curetting warts/verrucas or incising an abscess.

EMLA cream

EMLA cream is a topical anaesthetic cream containing lignocaine and prilocaine. Its main use is for children prior to cryocautery, venesection or injection. It should be left for at least an hour prior to the procedure. A useful strategy is to mark out the area to be anaesthetized and give the mother the cream to apply thickly and cover with an Opsite dressing or clingfilm at least an hour beforehand.

Other topical agents

For skin cleansing cetrimide solution is satisfactory, povidone–iodine being a skin antiseptic preferred by some. Topical antibiotics of use postoperatively include neomycin and bacitracin powder or oxytetracycline plus hydrocortisone spray. Chloramphenicol ointment is the favourite of some surgeons. Opsite is an invaluable protective dressing.

Anaphylaxis

This is dealt with in the chapter on resuscitation. A major reaction to the local anaesthetic is an ever-present, although very rare, possibility. Using too much local anaesthetic is a fault to avoid, and one should clearly take great care not to inject local anaesthetic directly into a blood vessel.

Wound infection

In some sites, such as the ingrowing toenail, postoperative infection is almost invariable (but rarely of major clinical significance). In the face infection can result in an unsightly wound and is a disaster.

To avoid infection:

- Do not neglect sterile technique.
- Prepare the site to be operated on properly.
- Do not operate on an infected site – if a sebaceous cyst is grossly infected, drain and treat with antibiotics to combat infection first, then operate at a later date.
- Choose your patients carefully – particularly beware those with an immune deficiency, diabetics and those with a poor circulation.
- Use good operative technique, avoiding haematomas, ragged skin edges or gaping suture lines.

The dangers of postoperative infection are possible systemic spread of the infection, poor wound healing and subsequent unsightly scars.

Bleeding

Bleeding can occur at any site, but is commoner in regions such as the scalp, face, ears, hands and scrotum. To avoid excessive bleeding:

- Use adrenaline with lignocaine where indicated (but once again, remember *never* to use adrenaline in the digits, nose, ears or penis).

- If possible, avoid operating on patients with a bleeding diathesis or who are on anticoagulants.
- Use good surgical technique, securing secondary haemostasis by using clips, cautery with a hyfrecator or hot wire, and by stitching bleeding vessels with an absorbable suture.

Note that a postoperative haematoma usually resolves satisfactorily with no need for intervention or antibiotics, although in certain situations (e.g. a

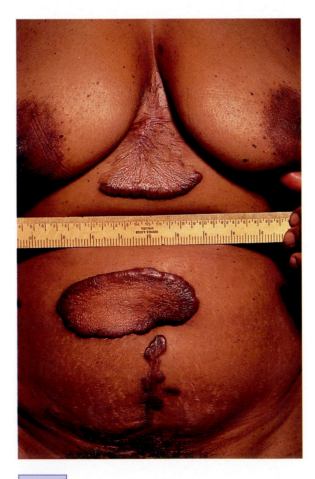

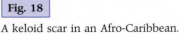

A keloid scar in an Afro-Caribbean.

large scrotal haematoma) evacuation may be required to prevent tissue necrosis.

Damage to surrounding structures

To avoid litigation it is essential to consider the underlying anatomy before attempting dissection.

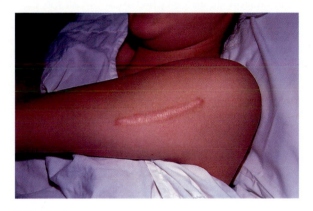

Fig. 19

A keloid scar in a Caucasian.

Damage to nerves can result in loss of function and anaesthesia. The facial nerve, for example, is clearly at risk to those operating deep in the facial territory. The key to success is to operate within your limitations, avoiding danger areas such as the face or palmar aspect of the hand.

Scars

Bad scars can be avoided by:

- Only operating along Langer's lines and skin creases
- Using appropriate blades and sutures, e.g. a 6/0 monofilament suture for the face
- Using a vertical incision, tension-free stitches and proper everting sutures
- Using subcuticular suturing to oppose the wound edges prior to skin suturing or the use of skin closure strips
- Taking care to avoid infection
- Being wary of certain patient groups, who scar easily. Afro-Caribbeans, for example, are susceptible to keloid scars. Examples of keloid scars are shown in Figures 18 and 19. The nipple-to-chin area is the commonest area for poor scarring. Before operating one could ask all patients how they scar.

8 Resuscitation in practice

All minor surgical procedures carry a risk, particularly when local anaesthetic is used. Acute anaphylaxis (with collapse, bronchospasm, laryngeal oedema and hypotension) is rare but well documented in this context. Bradycardia and hypoxia consequent to a faint is more commonly seen, and rarely patients may progress to a full tonic–clonic seizure. You must have the drugs and equipment for dealing with any such emergencies:

- A laryngoscope
- An endotracheal tube
- Airways (different sizes, including paediatric)
- An Ambubag and mask
- An intravenous line and cannulae
- Suction equipment
- Adrenaline injection (1 in 1000 and 1 in 10000)
- Aminophylline or salbutamol injections
- Atropine injection

- Calcium chloride injection
- Chlorpheniramine injection
- Hydrocortisone injection
- Rectal diazepam plus diazepam for intravenous injection
- Sodium bicarbonate 8.4% solution for injection.

Resuscitation kits can be purchased with all the equipment needed (Fig. 20). Make sure such a kit is readily available whenever you are undertaking minor surgery.

You should keep all the drugs required separately in a box (Fig. 21), with a designated member of the team being responsible for ensuring they are kept up to date. Taped to the box should be instructions on the dose of adrenaline to use by intramuscular injection in the case of acute anaphylaxis (see Table).

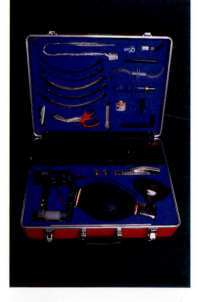

Fig. 20

A resuscitation kit.

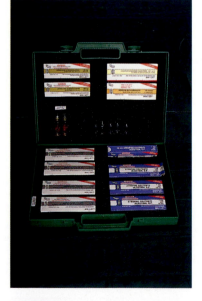

Fig. 21

A box of drugs for use in resuscitation.

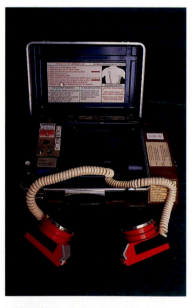

Fig. 22

A defibrillator.

Age	Dose of 1 in 1000 adrenaline
Less than 1 year	0.05 ml
1 year	0.1 ml
2 years	0.2 ml
3–4 years	0.3 ml
5 years	0.4 ml
6–12 years	0.5 ml
Over 12	0.5–1 ml

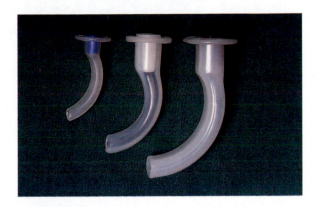

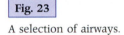

A selection of airways.

When dealing with anaphylaxis, first lay the patient flat in the recovery position then, provided the patient has not immediately recovered, administer adrenaline as above. The dose may be repeated 10 minutes later, according to response. Following adrenaline an injection of chlorpheniramine can be given, the dose for adults being 10 mg by slow intravenous, intramuscular or subcutaneous injection. Chlorpheniramine injection is not recommended for children. Intravenous corticosteroids are also of value (hydrocortisone 200 mg intravenously).

An ECG (electrocardiograph) should be available and a defibrillator (Fig. 22), and oxygen would complete a fully professional resuscitation kit. Although expensive, a defibrillator can save lives. Finally, remember to have a selection of airways of different sizes available (Fig. 23).

All those employed in a surgery should have had training in basic cardiopulmonary resuscitation (CPR). There should be a wallchart posted in the minor surgery room clearly detailing the steps in CPR. In particular, every team member should know how to put a patient in the recovery position – in the common case of a patient fainting, this is often all that is required.

Basic cardiopulmonary resuscitation

In a surgery setting the procedure will follow these seven basic steps:

1. Determine a patient's responsiveness by shaking the patient and shouting.

2. If there is no response, lay the patient supine and immediately call for help. The person who hears your call should immediately telephone for an ambulance plus paramedic to take the patient to hospital.

3. Without delay, open the patient's mouth and clear out any debris/vomit/loose teeth. The airway can be opened by the simple positioning of the patient's head – with the chin lifted upwards and the head tilted backwards (Fig. 24). This will prevent the tongue obstructing the airway – one of the commonest preventable disasters.

4. Determine the patient's breathing pattern and feel for a pulse. It should take only seconds to see if a patient is breathing (listening over the patient's mouth, watching the chest for breathing movements) and to check whether there is a carotid pulse or not.

5. If there is a carotid pulse present but no respiration, start artificial ventilation by mouth-to-mouth resuscitation or by using a mask. Note that

there has been no evidence that HIV infection can be acquired by mouth-to-mouth resuscitation. The technique is simple: you keep the patient in the open airway position described above (chin lifted and head tilted backwards), then pinch the patient's nose, opening his mouth fully and making a seal with your own (Fig. 25). As you exhale watch for the patient's chest moving. It may only take two or three ventilations to re-establish respiration.

6. If there is no carotid pulse you must start compressing the chest. Ensure that the patient is firmly on the floor, feel for the lower part of the sternum and interlock your hands with the heel of the first hand right up against the bone. Compression should be to a depth of 4–5 cm at a rate of 80 per minute. If you are attempting this alone, you should aim for 15 compressions to two artificial ventilations.

7. If signs of recovery are confirmed by breathing restarting and the presence of a carotid pulse, the patient can be placed in the recovery position (but still closely monitored until further help arrives).

The European Resuscitation Council have produced guidelines for advanced cardiac life support (Fig. 26).

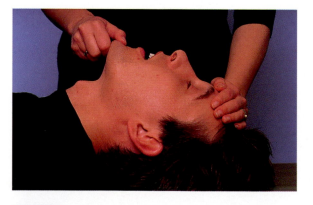

Fig. 24
Tilt head position.

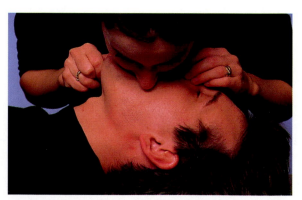

Fig. 25
Mouth-to-mouth resuscitation.

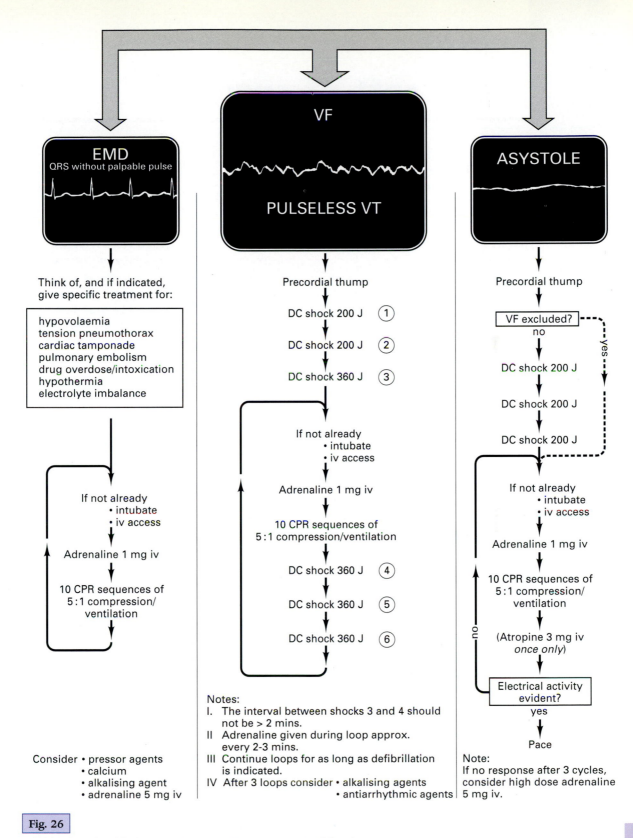

EMD
QRS without palpable pulse

VF

PULSELESS VT

ASYSTOLE

Think of, and if indicated,
give specific treatment for:

hypovolaemia
tension pneumothorax
cardiac tamponade
pulmonary embolism
drug overdose/intoxication
hypothermia
electrolyte imbalance

If not already
• intubate
• iv access

Adrenaline 1 mg iv

10 CPR sequences of
5:1 compression/
ventilation

Consider • pressor agents
• calcium
• alkalising agent
• adrenaline 5 mg iv

Precordial thump

DC shock 200 J ①

DC shock 200 J ②

DC shock 360 J ③

If not already
• intubate
• iv access

Adrenaline 1 mg iv

10 CPR sequences of
5:1 compression/ventilation

DC shock 360 J ④

DC shock 360 J ⑤

DC shock 360 J ⑥

Notes:
I. The interval between shocks 3 and 4 should
    not be > 2 mins.
II Adrenaline given during loop approx.
    every 2-3 mins.
III Continue loops for as long as defibrillation
    is indicated.
IV After 3 loops consider • alkalising agents
                          • antiarrhythmic agents

Precordial thump

VF excluded?   no

DC shock 200 J

DC shock 200 J

DC shock 200 J

yes

If not already
• intubate
• iv access

Adrenaline 1 mg iv

10 CPR sequences of
5:1 compression/
ventilation

(Atropine 3 mg iv
once only)

no

Electrical activity
evident?
yes

Pace

Note:
If no response after 3 cycles,
consider high dose adrenaline
5 mg iv.

Fig. 26

Advanced cardiac life support (European Resuscitation Guidelines).

17

The choice of suture material and the stitch used is dictated both by personal preference and the nature of the wound to be closed. Some simple rules that can be applied are as follows:

1. Always use the finest suture possible, e.g. 6/0 on the face and hands, 4/0 elsewhere.
2. Leave the suture in for as short a time as possible to avoid marking the skin, e.g. for 5 days on the face and up to 10 days on the back.
3. Where possible use subcutaneous and subcuticular suturing to avoid skin stitches. Steristrip skin closures can be used if no skin sutures are required.
4. Always use monofilament rather than braided suture to reduce the risk of tissue reaction.
5. A smear of antibiotic ointment over a wound may be used to reduce the risk of infection.

Types of suture illustrated are:

1. A plain suture (Fig. 27). This is the simplest of sutures and can be used where there is no underlying cavity, either in a simple superficial wound or where subcutaneous tissue has been previously brought together with a subcutaneous or fat suture. Always enter the skin with the needle at 90° to the skin and similarly exit with the needle at 90° to the skin. The knot should be triple tied and not too tight. For aesthetic reasons the knots should all be on the same side.

2. A subcutaneous suture (Fig. 28). The subcutaneous suture illustrated uses plain (undyed) Vicryl or Dexon. If used carefully the resultant wound is closed as a hairline, with no suture marks and no need to remove sutures. Care must be taken to ensure good approximation of the edges and the

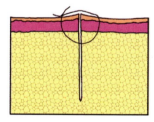

Fig. 27

A correctly positioned suture.

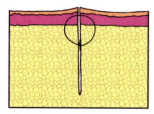

Fig. 28

A correctly positioned subcutaneous suture.

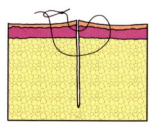

Fig. 29

A correctly positioned mattress suture.

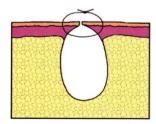

Fig. 30

An incorrectly fashioned suture, leaving a large dead space.

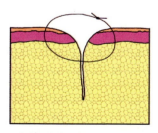

Fig. 31

A lax suture, leading to wide, slow-to-heal scars.

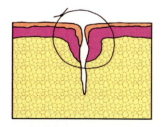

Fig. 32

Inverted wound edges – these will heal poorly.

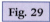

knots should always lie deep in the wound, as illustrated. Using a curved needle the suture is introduced into the subcutaneous fat, bringing the needle out just below the surface of the skin. The needle is reinserted into the corresponding point below the skin on the opposite side and brought out into the fatty layer. The knot is then tied in the fatty layer. This suture is now used preferentially in many situations.

3. The mattress suture (Fig. 29). This achieves both good approximation of the wound edges (by everting them) and obliteration of any potential space below the wound. Again, the needle entry and exit points should be at 90° to the skin. In large wounds alternating mattress and plain sutures can give very acceptable cosmetic results.

Figures 30–32 show examples of poor suture technique, which lead to poor scars with the potential for wound dehiscence and infection. Figures 33–36 illustrate the technique described on page 18 of closing a wound using a subcutaneous suture, with Steristrips rather than skin sutures completing the final closure.

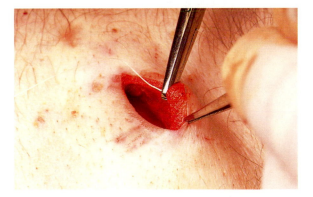

Fig. 33

Suture being applied from fat into subcutaneous tissue.

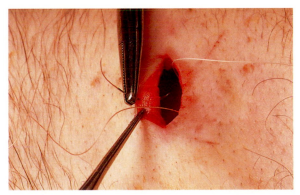

Fig. 34

Suture being applied from superficial to deep tissue.

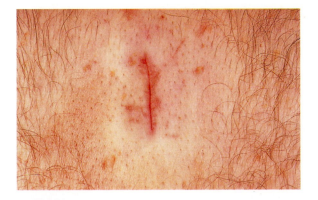

Fig. 35

Hairline wound left after closure.

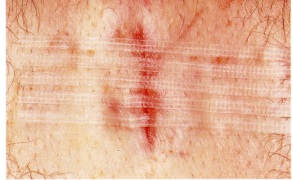

Fig. 36

Final closure reinforced by Steristrips.

Excising a sebaceous cyst

Sebaceous cysts are caused by blocked sebaceous ducts in sebaceous glands. The retained secretions cause the cyst to enlarge, and when the sac is opened the characteristic fatty or cheesy secretion confirms the diagnosis. Sebaceous cysts come in all sizes. They are usually solitary but may occasionally have daughter cysts.

The typical appearance of a sebaceous cyst usually makes the diagnosis. The key diagnostic feature to look for is the presence of a punctum. A sebaceous cyst may rarely be confused with such lesions as a lipoma, a vascular lesion in the scalp, a neurofibroma, a parotid tumour in the parotid area, a branchial cyst in the neck or a dermoid cyst. Dermoid cysts have no punctum and the overlying skin is adherent to the cyst.

Sebaceous cysts commonly occur on the back, scalp and ears. They can, however, occur in many other sites – even on the soles of the feet and palms of the hand. Beware of sebaceous cysts on the face or neck – these are the sites where confusion with other structures is more likely.

Reasons for removal

1. Size: a large cyst on the scalp could, for example, interfere with the patient combing their hair.

2. Cosmesis: many are removed because of their ugly appearance.
3. Infection: sebaceous cysts can become infected, forming an abscess.

In this case the abscess should be incised and drained, the patient prescribed oral antibiotics and the excision postponed until a later date.

Surgical principles when excising a sebaceous cyst

Figures 37–42 show excision of a preauricular sebaceous cyst – beware of operating at this site, as it is close to the facial nerve.

- As above, do not excise large infected cysts – drain and treat first.
- You must remove the wall of the cyst to avoid recurrence. Ideally the cyst should be excised intact.
- Careful infiltration of local anaesthetic may separate the superficial part of a cyst from the overlying skin.
- The usual approach is a vertical line of incision over the punctum site. With large cysts you may

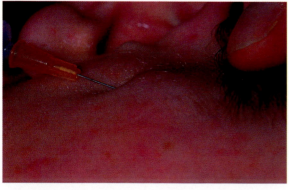

Fig. 37

Infiltration of local anaesthetic over the site.

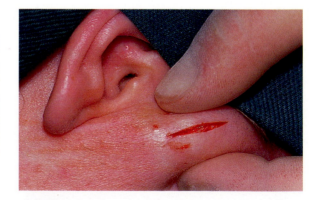

Fig. 38

Incision over the punctum site down to the capsule.

need to excise an ellipse of skin over the cyst to facilitate skin closure.
- The incision is carried down to the capsule, followed by dissection around the capsule with mosquito forceps or fine scissors.
- If you do puncture the cyst, ensure that you remove the wall by catching it with artery forceps and gently teasing it loose.
- With a large cyst you may need to use an

absorbable suture to obliterate the remaining cavity.
- Closure may be achieved using interrupted Prolene sutures, but a mattress suture can be used to good effect to obliterate a large space.
- Use 6/0 sutures if operating on the face, 4/0 elsewhere. The sutures should be removed after 5 days on the face and neck, 7–8 days on the scalp and up to 10 days on the trunk.

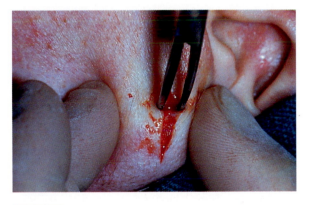

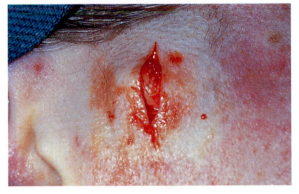

Fig. 39

Blunt dissection with mosquito forceps to further expose the capsule.

Fig. 40

Capsule visible in the base of the wound.

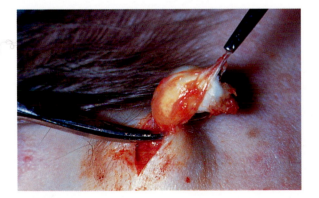

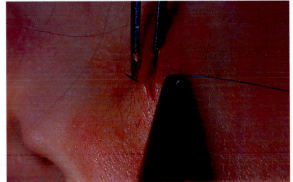

Fig. 41

Blunt and sharp dissection to remove the capsule intact (**NB:** dissect close to the capsule).

Fig. 42

A 6/0 Prolene suture closes the wound.

Excising a lipoma

Lipomas are benign fatty tumours which can occur in various tissue planes, from relatively superficial in the subcutaneous tissue to deep below and attached to fascia, to more retroperitoneal positions. They can grow to a considerable size and are usually encapsulated, but may occur in a multilobulated form with fibrous bands matting the lipoma to the underlying tissue. There is a limited potential for malignant change and rarely a lipoma may calcify. A few patients will have multiple lipomas and this may be familial. Dercum's disease is a specific disorder characterized by multiple lipomas.

The common soft fatty tumour lying in subcutaneous tissue presents little problem, but deeper lipomas can be mistaken for other lesions. Differential diagnosis will include a fibroadenoma, a neurofibroma, a sebaceous cyst and vascular lesions. Lipomas can occur anywhere in the body, including the scalp, face, hands and back.

Reasons for removal

1. Size: some lipomas can become very large and necessitate removal on size grounds alone.

2. Pressure effects: if the lipoma is pressing on surrounding structures and thus causing symptoms.
3. Cosmesis: as with sebaceous cysts.

Surgical principles when excising a lipoma

Figures 43–48 show the excision of a lipoma from the midline of the back – beware of excising at this site as lipomas in this position can extend deeply.

- Do not try to remove very large lipomas, e.g. in the buttock. Large lipomas (which may extend to deeper tissues) are best left for hospital excision. Lipomas in the midline of the back often extend deeply, and are best avoided by less experienced surgeons. The face is another area in which to exercise caution, because of (a) the possibility of facial nerve damage while attempting removal and (b) the possibility of a poor cosmetic result. Lipomas on the face are best left to plastic surgeons. Finally, a lipoma in the axilla or hands is one to refer to a specialist, again because of the possibility of damaging underlying structures.

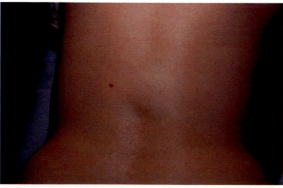

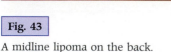

Fig. 43

A midline lipoma on the back.

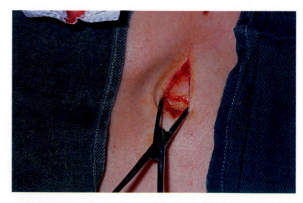

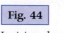

Fig. 44

Incision down to the capsule, widened with blunt dissection.

- You must try and remove a lipoma whole or there is a good chance that it will recur.
- You can gauge how deep a lipoma is situated by trying to pick up the skin over it: if both skin and superficial fat can be separated from the lipoma it will be a deep one, but if only the skin lifts the lipoma is superficially situated and ideal for minor surgery.
- You may need to infiltrate local anaesthetic into deeper tissue planes if your dissection carries you that far.
- After removal of a lipoma you may be left with a large hole. First ensure that there is no residual bleeding (by ligation or cautery) and then obliterate the dead space by suturing before closing the wound with a 4/0 suture (4/0 assumes you are not operating on the face).

You may not need to dissect a small lipoma out. In certain sites (the forearm, for example) it may be possible to incise above the lipoma and, by squeezing the surrounding skin, scoop it out with your gloved finger. This technique is illustrated in Figs 49–52.

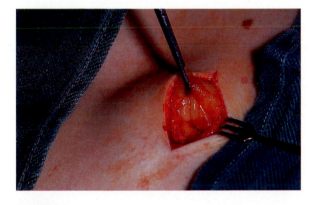

Fig. 45

Lipoma grasped with forceps to enable further blunt and sharp dissection.

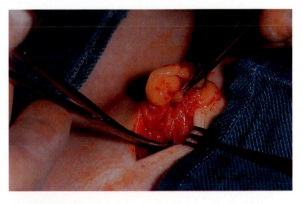

Fig. 46

Slow mobilization of the lipoma.

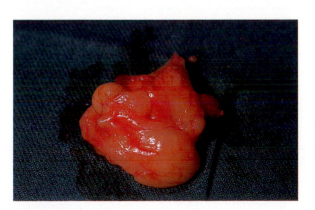

Fig. 47

Excised lipoma (intact).

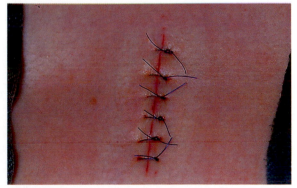

Fig. 48

Closure of the wound with 4/0 Prolene.

Excising a lipoma

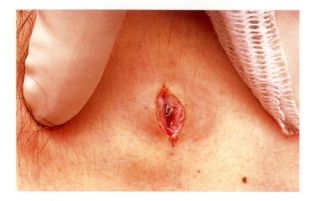

Fig. 49

Incision down to the capsule.

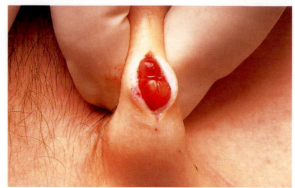

Fig. 50

Exerting gentle sideways pressure.

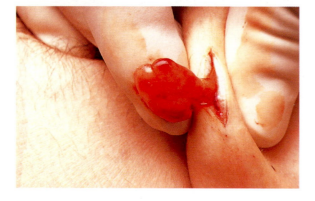

Fig. 51

Lipoma extruding from underlying tissues.

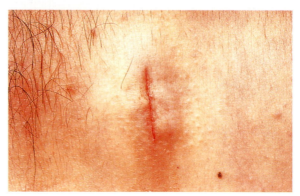

Fig. 52

Closure with subcuticular undyed Vicryl.

13 Excising an ingrowing toenail

An ingrowing toenail is caused by a nail edge penetrating deeply into the surrounding tissue, with resultant inflammation, infection and pain. It has a variety of causes, most notably pressure from incorrect footwear, improper cutting of toenails (short and rounded rather than straight) and infection. Ingrowing toenails are commonest in young adults.

The diagnosis is evident from the appearance. There is often considerable secondary infection and granulation tissue. The big toe is the most commonly affected, but an ingrowing toenail can occur in any toe.

Reasons for excision are pain and infection. Without intervention the situation will worsen.

Surgical principles when excising an ingrowing toenail

- At the earliest stage use of a cottonwool pledget to separate the nail from the damaged surrounding tissue may be successful. However, in the vast majority of cases surgery is required.
- An improperly treated toenail, removing portions of the nail rather than a formal resection, will result in more problems than if the nail had been left alone.
- Ingrowing toenails tend to recur even after operation. Postoperatively explain to the patient the basics of good nail care (comfortable shoes, correct nail cutting, etc.).
- Infection in the surrounding tissue is the rule rather than the exception in the case of ingrowing toenails, and does not preclude operation. Prior treatment with antibiotics is not usually required unless the toenail is grossly infected.
- For anaesthesia a ring block of 1% lignocaine is recommended, as outlined below. *Never use Adrenaline.*
  Technique of a ring block:
  (i) First clean the skin with cetrimide.

(ii) For a tourniquet there are two useful options: using catheter rubber tubing with a clip or using the finger portion of a surgical glove. With the latter the technique is to place the finger of the glove over the toe, cut the tip of the glove off and then roll the glove proximally along the toe. This will then exsanguinate the digit as well as acting as a tourniquet.

(iii) Using an orange 25 G $\times \frac{5}{8}$ in needle, infiltrate 1 ml of 1% plain lignocaine into the dorsum of the toe over the extensor tendon. Then advance the needle through the anaesthetized area to the lateral and medial borders of the toe, infiltrating the digital nerves on either side with 2 ml of 1% plain lignocaine. Finally, the needle may be advanced from this dorsal position further to infiltrate any plantar nerve supply to the toe.

(iv) Allow at least 10 minutes to ensure adequate anaesthesia before beginning to operate.

(v) Always remember to remove the tourniquet at the end of the operation!

- There are various techniques used to manage ingrowing toenails. In family practice the preferred technique is a wedge resection (Figs 53–64). Total nail ablation, removing the complete germinal matrix (a formal Zadek's procedure), may occasionally be required for a recurrent ingrowing toenail and this procedure is illustrated in Figures 65–72. Finally, many surgeons advocate the use of phenol, and phenolization will also be discussed (Figs 73–80).

Illustrated in Figures 59–64 are the final stages of the wedge resection of an ingrowing toenail. Note that it is essential to remove the tourniquet (especially if using rubber bands or the finger portion of a surgical glove) before applying the dressing. Routine postoperative antibiotics are not necessary.

Excising an ingrowing toenail

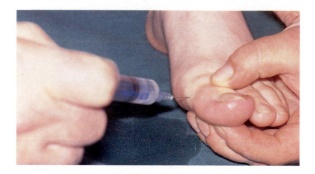

Fig. 53

Instilling a ring block: infiltration of 1% lignocaine *without* adrenaline.

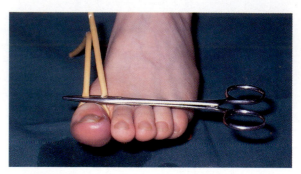

Fig. 54

Applying a tourniquet (in this case catheter tubing).

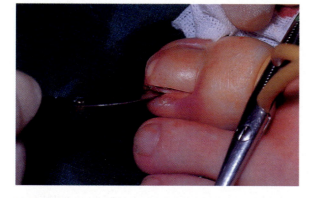

Fig. 55

Incising through the nail and nailbed.

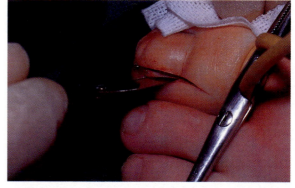

Fig. 56

Extending the excision into the germinal matrix.

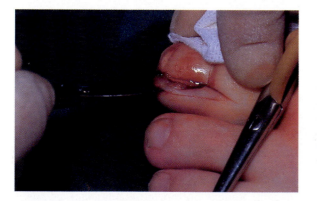

Fig. 57

Further excision to remove a wedge of nail and granulomatous tissue.

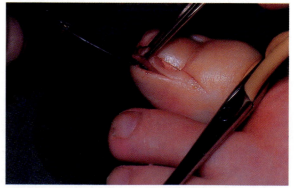

Fig. 58

Lifting the nail segment and dissecting out the nailbed.

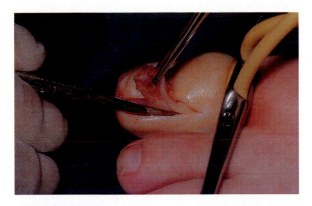

Fig. 59

Dissection to ensure that the germinal matrix is completely excised.

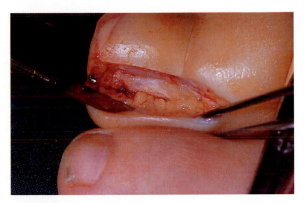

Fig. 60

The wedge of tissue has now been removed.

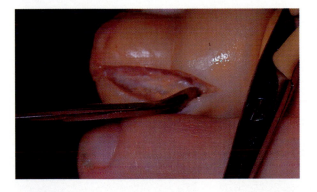

Fig. 61

Curettage to ensure there is no residual matrix.

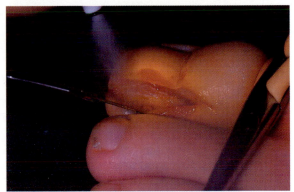

Fig. 62

Application of a topical spray (in this case povidone–iodine).

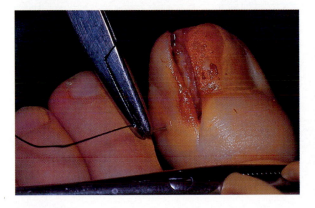

Fig. 63

Suture of the angular portion of the wound.

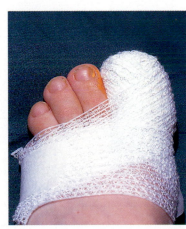

Fig. 64

Following suture apply an adequate firm dressing (be sure you have removed any tourniquet first).

Zadek's procedure

Zadek's procedure is the procedure of total nail ablation, removing the complete germinal matrix. It is not something to be undertaken lightly and its main use is for those with recurrently ingrowing toenails or those with onychogryphosis (see p. 32). Patient selection is important. One would generally try two wedge resections before terming an ingrowing toenail 'recurrent' and worthy of consideration for a Zadek's procedure.

It is important to emphasize to the patient at the outset that the procedure will result in a permanent lack of a toenail – some will mistakenly believe that the nail will regrow. When counselled in this manner, some patients will decline the procedure (demonstrating once again the value of a comprehensive discussion about any operation with the patient before surgery is commenced). The patient should also be warned that the nailbed may be tender for a few months after the procedure.

Complications

As regards the complications of a Zadek's procedure, four are worth noting:

1. Sepsis – as with any toenail surgery.
2. Osteomyelitis of the terminal phalanx due to an inappropriately aggressive technique traumatizing the bone.
3. Ischaemia of the toe due to too much pressure on the bandage (or the use of adrenaline).
4. Recurrence due to poor technique.

The technique itself is relatively straightforward and is illustrated in Figures 65–72. Because ingrowing toenails are so common, it is certainly a technique worth adding to your surgical repertoire. Figures 69–72 illustrate the final stages of the Zadek's procedure.

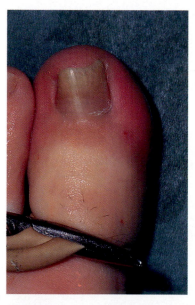

Fig. 65

The ingrowing toenail.

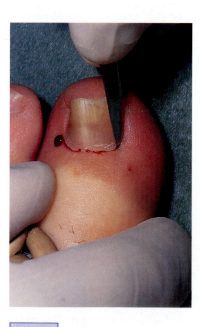

Fig. 66

The incision of the nail margin.

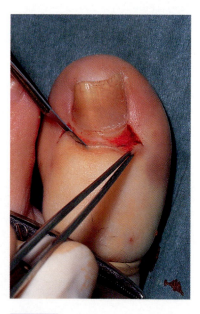

Fig. 67

Reflecting the flap proximally.

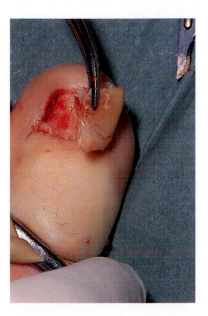

Fig. 68

The nail lifted clear.

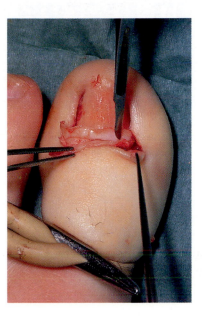

Fig. 69

Excision of the germinal matrix.

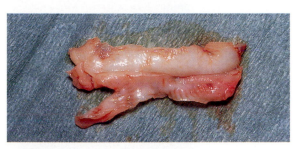

Fig. 70

The intact germinal matrix as removed.

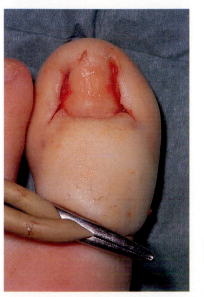

Fig. 71

The clean nailbed.

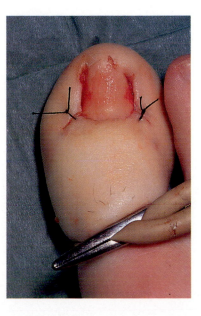

Fig. 72

Angular sutures. Following suturing the wound is dressed as for the wedge excision.

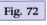

14 Phenolization of an ingrowing toenail

Phenolization is an alternative to wedge excision of an ingrowing toenail. The chemical destruction of the germinal matrix using phenol has been advocated by many as the treatment of choice. This technique's advantages and disadvantages compared with wedge excision are:

Advantages:

- Less destructive of tissue
- Less painful than wedge excision
- Bleeding less of a problem
- Secondary infection less of a problem
- Can be performed if infection present.

Disadvantages:

- If you fail to neutralize the phenol properly you can get significant tissue damage and poor wound healing.
- If phenol spills on to normal tissue (either the patient's or the surgeon's) it will burn the skin badly.
- If you use insufficient phenol for too short a time, the germinal matrix is not destroyed and recurrence will occur.

Principles of phenolization of the ingrowing toenail

- Always wear gloves to protect your skin from a phenol burn. Protect the patient's surrounding tissue with petroleum jelly, for example.
- Use a freshly prepared 80% phenol solution, *not* the oily 5% phenol injection used for injecting haemorrhoids.
- Prior to phenolization, completely remove part of the nail edge down to the germinal matrix, ensuring that no fragments of nail remain – phenol cannot work through nail remnants.
- Ensure adequate phenolization, neutralizing with alcohol after 3 minutes to ensure no further tissue destruction.
- Following neutralization of the phenol the toe is dressed (for example, with petroleum jelly gauze) and checked 24 hours later. The toe is dressed daily as required, and should be comfortable for most activities after a week.

Figures 73–80 illustrate the technique of phenolization of the ingrowing toenail. Figures 77–80 are the final steps.

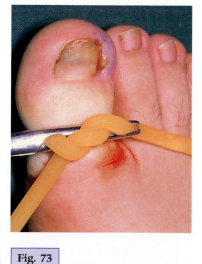

Fig. 73

Tourniquet applied to the great toe.

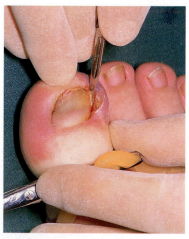

Fig. 74

Incision of the nail laterally.

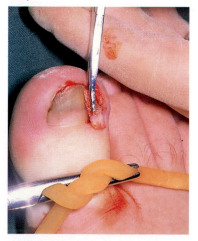

Fig. 75

Fragment of nail avulsed.

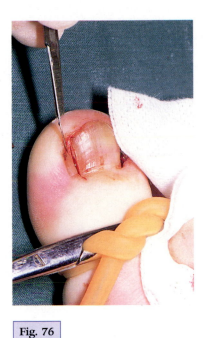

Fig. 76

Medial side of nail incised and avulsed.

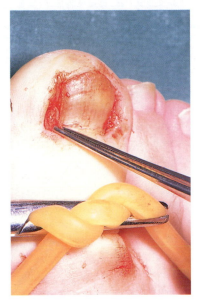

Fig. 77

Resulting cavity cleared of cellular debris.

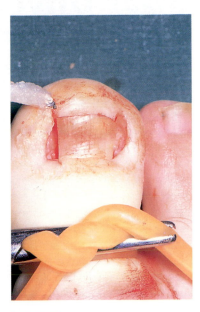

Fig. 78

Surrounding tissue protected with petroleum jelly.

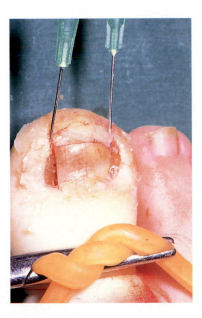

Fig. 79

A pledget of cotton wool is wrapped around a green needle, soaked in phenol and applied to the germinal matrix for 3 minutes.

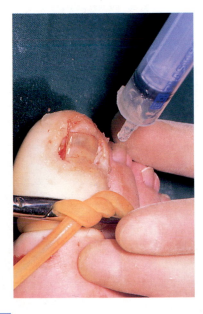

Fig. 80

Phenol neutralized with saline or alcohol.

31

15 Onychogryphosis

A commonly seen condition (Figs 81, 82), especially in the elderly, where there is an excessive and permanent irregular thickening of the nail. Chiropodists treat the minor cases but many cases will need surgery. Removing the nail by itself has a high recurrence rate, so the surgical treatment of choice is a Zadek's procedure along the lines already described for the ingrowing toenail. In some patients – the elderly with poor peripheral circulation, diabetics with poor wound healing or where there is sepsis – removing the nail may, however, be the appropriate course of action. In the case of sepsis a definitive operation can follow once the nail has been removed and the sepsis drained. Some surgeons favour phenolization of the nailbed following nail removal, but to successfully prevent recurrence we would still recommend a formal Zadek's nailbed ablation.

Technique for removal of the nail

1. After cleansing the site with cetrimide anaesthetize with a ring block, as described in the section on excising an ingrowing toenail. *Do not use adrenaline with the lignocaine.*

2. Once the ring block is in place and working, insert a mosquito clip under the nail. Open the blades to separate the nail from the bed.
3. Grasp the nail with heavy forceps (e.g. Spencer Wells forceps) and twist to free the edge of the nail from the nailfolds. Further gentle traction should avulse the nail from the underlying skin. Bleeding is usually minimal with this procedure.
4. Clean loose skin from the wound.
5. Dress with a Sofratuille dressing.
6. Bandage the foot. Dressings should be changed daily for 7 days.

For a Zadek's procedure see page 28.

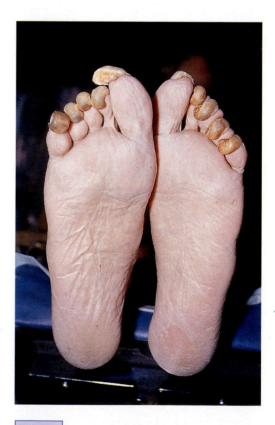

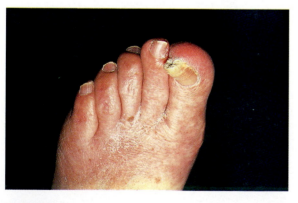

Fig. 81

Onychogryphosis of the nail.

Fig. 82

A plantar view.

16 Excising skin lesions

There are many skin lesions that are suitable for excision. The commonest lesions excised in minor surgery sessions are:

- Skin tags, papillomas, seborrhoeic warts
- Keratoacanthomas
- Skin naevi
- Histiocytomas
- Fibromas
- Calcifying epitheliomas
- Small skin lesions requiring diagnosis.

Many skin lesions can be either cauterized or excised. Skin naevi are best excised (Fig. 83); verrucas are best cauterized. Electrocautery is used by some for skin tags, papillomas and simple warts.

The diagnosis is usually obvious but beware the undiagnosed pigmented lesion (see below). Keratoacanthomas can easily be confused with squamous cell carcinomas. Small basal cell carcinomas (BCC) can be removed from the face as a minor surgery procedure, although skin closure can be difficult with larger BCCs, requiring hospital referral.

Skin lesions can occur anywhere on the body, certain ones having a preference for certain sites, e.g. histiocytomas on the legs.

Reasons for removal

There are three main reasons: (i) cosmetic, where the appearance is unsightly; (ii) where the lesion is irritating, rubbing on clothes or a strapline; (iii) for diagnosis.

Surgical principles when excising skin lesions

- First consider the differential diagnosis. If there is any suggestion of the possibility of a malignant melanoma do not proceed, and refer the patient urgently to a dermatologist.
- Before excising the lesion infiltrate widely with local anaesthetic (Fig. 84). Wait 5 minutes before beginning the excision procedure.

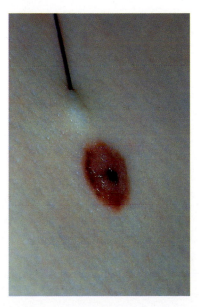

Fig. 83

A halo naevus on the trunk.

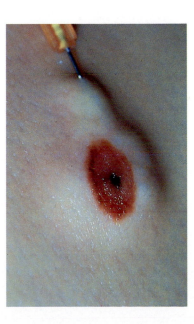

Fig. 84

Wide infiltration with 1% lignocaine plus adrenaline.

33

Excising skin lesions

- Use sterile technique and good surgical craft to avoid unsightly scar formation. Where possible, make your incision in the line of a skin crease (Figs 85, 86).
- Send all excised skin lesions for histology.
- Good skin closure is very important: close with 6/0 monofilament (Ethilon or Prolene) on the face, 4/0 monofilament elsewhere. If you are left with a gaping open wound approximate the skin edges first with 4/0 catgut or undyed Vicryl prior to skin closure.

- Following suturing some surgeons apply topical antibiotics such as chloramphenicol ointment before applying the dry dressing.
- Remove sutures after 5 days on the face, 7–10 days elsewhere.

The technique of excision biopsy of a skin lesion is fully detailed on page 66. Figures 87–90 illustrate the final steps in the surgical removal of a naevus.

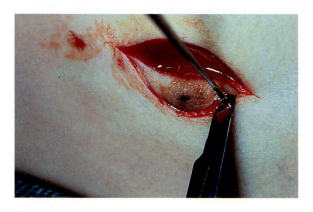

Fig. 85

An elliptical incision.

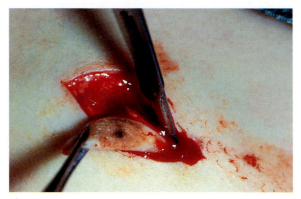

Fig. 86

Sharp dissection into the fatty layer and removal of the naevus.

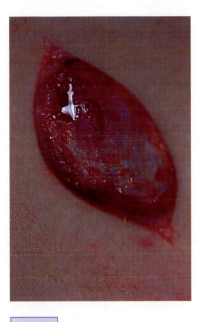

Fig. 87

A clear deficit following removal of the naevus.

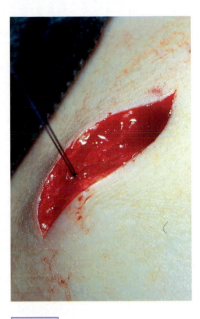

Fig. 88

Use of a subcutaneous Vicryl suture.

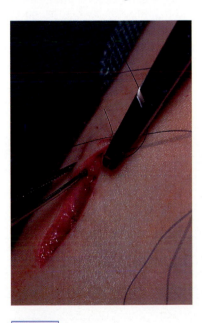

Fig. 89

Closure of the site with continuous Prolene.

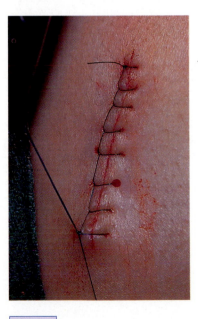

Fig. 90

The completed operation.

Cauterizing warts, verrucas and other lesions

Warts, which are caused by viruses, are part of the staple diet of minor surgery. There are as many different treatment protocols as there are sites for the warts. Plantar warts (verrucas) are perhaps the commonest type of wart presented to the family practitioner, and here the most-used alternatives are (1) use of a salicylic acid paint, rubbing the verruca with a pumice stone or manicure emery paper prior to the nightly application; (2) curettage under anaesthetic, with or without subsequent cautery to the base of the wart; (3) cryocautery. Except in very young children, where cryocautery may not be complied with, the cryocautery alternative is favoured. Cryocautery can also be used for hand warts, anogenital warts, skin tags, papillomas, solar keratoses, benign naevi and molluscum contagiosum. Paring warts down prior to cryocautery may lead to a more successful outcome. Seborrhoeic warts are often easier curetted.

The technique of cryocautery

There are several ways of performing cryocautery. The easiest is using simple cottonwool buds dipped in liquid nitrogen. Unfortunately this technique rarely freezes to a depth sufficient for proper treatment, only freezing to a depth of about 2mm. Clearly, you will have to have a fresh supply of liquid nitrogen available on the day you have your cryocautery clinic. An alternative method is to use an aerosol-based system such as the Histofreezer, which delivers a jet of solvent into a cottonwool bud. Again, this method is only suitable for superficial lesions. By far the most satisfactory method is to purchase a liquid nitrogen cryoprobe/cryospray, which will produce the consistently good results, with the required depth of penetration of the lesion, that will make it an invaluable addition to your minor surgery kit. Figures 91–94 illustrate the use of a cryoprobe. Lubricating jelly (KY jelly) is applied to the lesion to give good contact with the probe. Children find cryocautery more unpleasant,

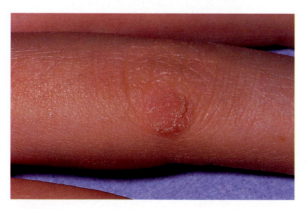

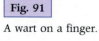

A wart on a finger.

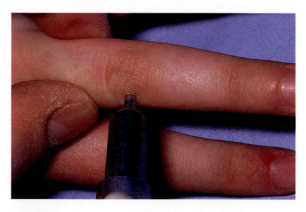

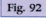

The Cryojet blunt probe applied (with KY jelly between the probe and finger). Apply for two freeze–thaw cycles.

and in children we would use EMLA cream as a local anaesthetic 1 hour before the cryocautery (the mother can apply it at home before bringing the child to the clinic).

Patients undergoing cryocautery should be given an information leaflet outlining the procedure (and what to expect afterwards) detailing the fact that some tingling/pain may be felt hours after the cryocautery; the fact that redness, blistering and swelling are to be expected and that the lesion will scab over in about a week.

Large verrucas may be quite resistant to treatment, needing multiple applications.

The technique of electrocautery

The technique of electrocautery (also more colourfully known as 'hot-wire cautery') is another useful addition to the armamentarium of those carrying out minor surgery. As the description suggests, the technique employs a red-hot wire to cut through and coagulate tissue.

Electrocautery is available in many forms, from a disposable battery-operated kit to a rechargeable device to more sophisticated mains-operated equipment (which will need regular checks from an electrician to guard against potential electrocution!).

This technique is the cheapest form of cautery, is simple, safe and easy to use, and leaves good scars. It must always be used with local anaesthesia, except for the tiniest of lesions. Its coagulating effect will stem bleeding, making it particularly useful for removing pedunculated lesions, skin tags or papillomas, where you can not only remove the lesion but also secure haemostasis by applying hot-wire cautery to the base.

One must clearly exercise due care that any neighbouring skin or structures are not burnt by the hot wire (e.g. if applying near a joint). Finally, one must still remember the cardinal principle of sending skin lesions for histology: simple skin tags and papillomas are readily identifiable and safe to cauterize, but if there is any doubt clearly you should not destroy unidentified lesions by electrocautery.

Figures 95–98 illustrate electrocautery to remove a small haemangioma.

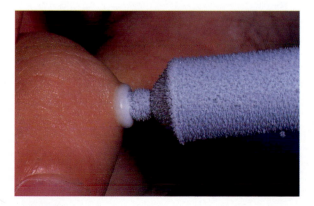

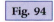
Fig. 93

An adequate ice ball.

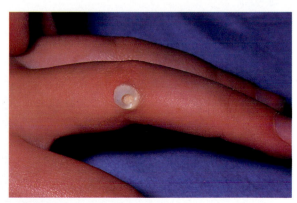

Fig. 94

A halo of frozen tissue around the lesion (**NB**: care must be taken not to freeze into the joint).

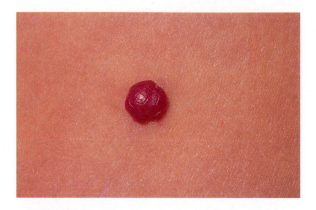

Fig. 95

A small haemangioma.

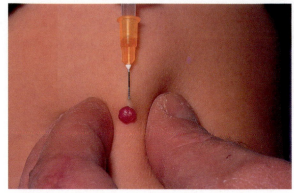

Fig. 96

Infiltration with local anaesthetic.

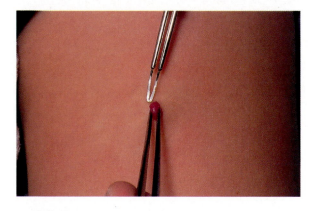

Fig. 97

The lesion grasped with forceps, with hot-wire cautery applied to the base to remove the lesion.

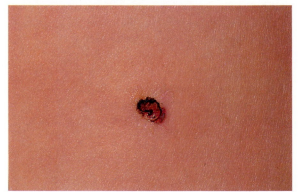

Fig. 98

The resulting small burn, the lesion having been removed.

18 Excising a ganglion

A ganglion is a gelatinous cyst connecting with a tendon sheath or joint capsule. This communication with the underlying tendon sheath/joint is important because it means that dissection and excision is not straightforward, owing to the attachment to deeper underlying structures, and that pressing, injecting or trying to aspirate the ganglion will usually result in recurrence as the cyst refills from below.

A ganglion has a characteristic smooth, jelly-like feel and this consistency, together with its occurrence in a typical site, generally makes the diagnosis an easy one.

The two most common sites for a ganglion are the dorsum of the wrist or foot (Fig. 99). They can, however, occur in relation to any joint or tendon sheath, including the flexor sheaths of the fingers.

Reasons for removal

Being entirely innocent structures, small ganglia causing no symptoms can be left alone. Some will resolve spontaneously. Large ganglia causing pressure symptoms owing to their size or unacceptable cosmetic appearance can be excised.

Surgical principles when excising a ganglion (Figs 100–102)

- Before surgery discuss the benign nature of ganglia with the patient, the pros and cons of removal, and the fact that there is always a possibility of recurrence despite your best efforts.
- Only ganglia on the dorsum of the foot or hand are eligible for local anaesthetic minor surgery – ganglia at other sites are best left for the specialist surgeon.
- Revise your anatomy before operating – you may be operating in a field containing important vessels and nerves!
- Aspiration or injection with steroids have a higher recurrence rate and are much less effective than surgical excision.

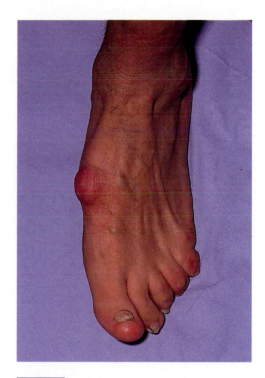

Fig. 99

A ganglion in the dorsum of the foot.

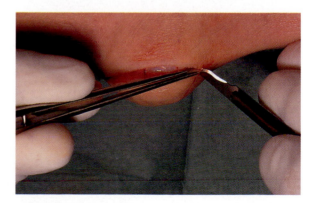

Fig. 100

Having infiltrated adequately with local anaesthetic, the primary incision is made over the ganglion to remove surplus skin.

39

Excising a ganglion

- Make sure you excise the wall of the ganglion completely and that you meticulously dissect the ganglion down to its origin at the tendon sheath or joint capsule, closing the resulting deficit with absorbable sutures.

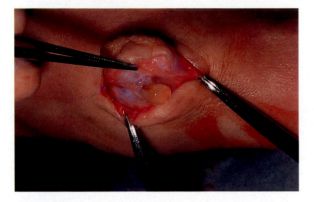

Fig. 101

Ganglion excised intact by careful dissection. Note the leakage of gelatinous material typical of a ganglion.

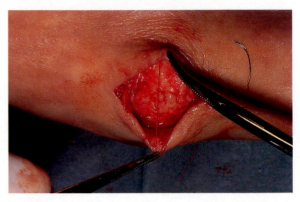

Fig. 102

Once excised, the cavity left can be sutured with Vicryl.

19 The ten principles of joint injection

1. **Make an accurate diagnosis** First make an accurate diagnosis of the presenting clinical condition: is it one which will respond to steroid injection therapy? Fully examine the joint and surrounding joints/tissues to confirm your diagnosis before injecting. An X-ray may be necessary.

2. **Revise your knowledge of the local anatomy before injecting** Before injecting ensure that you are fully aware of the surrounding nerves, tendons and blood vessels. You may wish to mark the site for injection prior to inserting the needle.

3. **Use aseptic non-touch technique** Wash and dry your hands thoroughly, cleanse the skin scrupulously with cetrimide or a spirit-based swab, use sterile syringes and needles, and only use single-dose vials of steroids/local anaesthetics. Use one needle to draw up the preparation being used and a new, clean, needle for the injection itself.

4. **Use the correct size of needle** This will depend on the size of the joint, e.g. a 21-gauge (21 G × $1\frac{1}{2}$ in green) needle for a shoulder injection but a 25-gauge (25 G × $\frac{5}{8}$ in orange) needle for a trigger finger. See individual injections.

5. **Use the correct preparation** Two long-acting depot steroid preparations are recommended – methylprednisolone acetate or triamcinolone hexacetonide. These are generally used for joint injection; for some soft tissue injections the shorter-acting hydrocortisone injection may be preferred. The steroid injection can be thoroughly mixed with the local anaesthetic lignocaine in the same syringe prior to injection. This will give immediate pain relief, but the patient should be warned that the local anaesthetic effect wears off in about 2 hours.

The correct amount of steroid and anaesthetic should be used, more volume being needed for larger joints (see specific injections).

6. **Observe contraindications to steroid injection**
- Do not inject an infected joint.
- Do not inject a patient suffering from a systemic infection.
- Do not inject fractured or unstable joints.
- Do not inject joints containing foreign bodies/prostheses.
- Do not inject the joints/tissues of patients with bleeding disorders or those on anticoagulants.
- Do not inject those who are significantly immunosuppressed.
- Do not inject those with a previous hypersensitivity to the injection material.
- Exercise caution with weight-bearing joints (hips, knees, ankles).

7. **Warn the patient after the injection**
- That pain may be worse or unaffected for 24–48 hours after the injection until the steroid begins to work
- Of the importance of reporting back any complications, including redness, heat or swelling of the joint, or other signs of possible infection (e.g. pyrexia).

Diabetics should be warned that steroid injections may destabilize their diabetes for 3–4 days.

8. **Wait at least 3–4 weeks between injections** It is wise not to repeat steroid injections within a month. Limit injections of a particular joint/soft tissue to three a year.

9. **Be alert to the complications of steroid injections**

- Infection
- Damage to nerves, tendons (including tendon rupture), blood vessels
- Local skin atrophy
- Skin depigmentation
- Tissue/joint damage as a result of repeated injection
- Systemic absorption of the steroid – rarely a problem but may destabilize a patient's diabetic control for 3–4 days.

10. **Know your limitations** Only perform procedures you are fully confident of performing correctly. If you are unsure about an injection do not attempt it!

20

Injecting the shoulder joint

Conditions to inject include rotator cuff syndrome/supraspinatus tendinitis/subacromial bursitis, adhesive capsulitis (frozen shoulder) and acromioclavicular joint subluxation.

Making the diagnosis

Rotator cuff syndrome/supraspinatus tendinitis/subacromial bursitis are all conditions producing the characteristic painful arc syndrome on abducting the shoulder. They usually respond to a subacromial bursa injection.

Adhesive capsulitis starts with an increasingly painful stiff joint, progressing to a phase where the stiffness is more prominent than the pain. There is a characteristic limitation of rotation as well as abduction, giving rise to the term 'frozen shoulder'. Capsulitis requires injection of the glenohumeral joint.

Acromioclavicular joint subluxation presents as pain and tenderness at the acromioclavicular joint. It is a common sports injury and an X-ray will be helpful in confirming the diagnosis.

Before injection confirm any limited/painful abduction and/or rotation of the shoulder joint and take a proper history. Beware of referred pain, especially from the neck – test neck movements, biceps reflexes and for shoulder-tip anaesthesia to exclude any neck pathology. Remember other conditions causing a painful shoulder, including polymyalgia rheumatica, septic or rheumatoid arthritis and gout. Acute presentations of shoulder pain may be related to heart/lung conditions. If at all in doubt, organize relevant tests. If the picture is not a classic one the shoulder is a joint worth X-raying – in particular, the shoulder is a common site for metastases. Remember that diabetes may present initially with shoulder pain – test the urine!

Needle and preparation to use

Use a 21-gauge (21 G $\times$ 1$\frac{1}{2}$ in green) needle. For the subacromial bursa use 2–3 ml of 1% lignocaine mixed with 1 ml (40 mg) methylprednisolone. For the glenohumeral joint you need a larger volume – 5 ml of 1% lignocaine plus 40 mg of methylprednislone. For the acromioclavicuar joint use 0.5 ml of 1% lignocaine plus 40 mg methylprednisolone.

Injection technique

- For the subacromial bursa identify the tip of the acromion and palpate the space between the acromion and the head of the humerus. This space, just below the acromion, can be marked with a fingernail prior to swabbing the skin. Injection should be easy, entering laterally and sliding the needle just under the tip of the acromion into the bursa (Fig. 103) without meeting bony resistance.
- The posterolateral approach is the easiest option for the glenohumeral joint (Fig. 104). Identify the spine of the scapula and follow it to the point where it angulates to form the acromion. About 2 cm below and medial to this point should be the site of needle entry, inserting with the needle pointing in the direction of the sternoclavicular joint. The needle is advanced slowly until you feel the give as it enters the joint through the posterior joint capsule (Fig. 105). If bone is encountered withdraw slightly and reposition the needle.
- Inject the acromioclavicular joint directly into the joint, which is located at the distal end of the clavicle (Fig. 106).

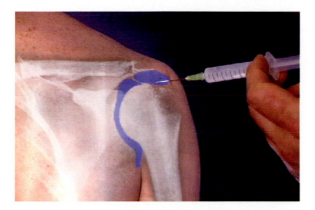

Fig. 103

Schematic representation showing the injection of steroid into the subacromial bursa.

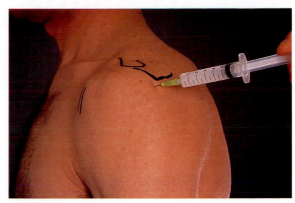

Fig. 104

The posterolateral approach to the shoulder joint.

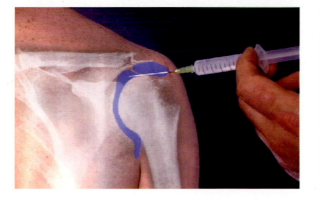

Fig. 105

Schematic representation showing an injection of steroid into the glenohumeral joint.

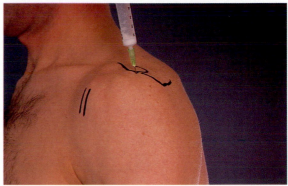

Fig. 106

The acromioclavicular joint being injected with steroid. There are a wide variety of joint conditions that respond to steroid injection therapy.

21

Injecting a bicipital tendinitis

Bicipital tendinitis presents as pain/tenderness in the bicipital groove and responds well to local injection. Use a 21-gauge (21 G × $1\frac{1}{2}$ in green) needle and 2–3 ml of 1% lignocaine mixed with 1 ml (40 mg) methylprednisolone.

Injection technique

Locate the bicipital groove and insert the needle along it, entering from above downwards (Figs 107, 108) and injecting the tender area. The injection flow should be smooth, without any resistance – if it does not flow easily withdraw and reinject. Do *not* inject under pressure – there is a real danger of tendon rupture if you inject the tendon itself, so care should always be exercised when performing this procedure.

A course of physiotherapy is useful after the injection.

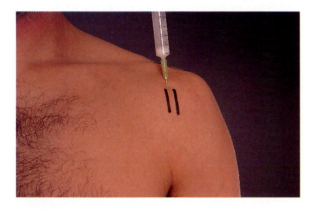

Fig. 107

Injecting a bicipital tendinitis.

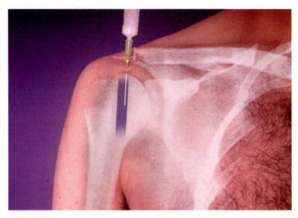

Fig. 108

Schematic representation showing an injection into the bicipital groove for bicipital tendinitis.

22 Injecting a tennis or golfer's elbow

Tennis elbow is a straightforward diagnosis, presenting with pain and localized tenderness over the lateral epicondyle at the site of the common extensor origin. The diagnosis can be confirmed by eliciting pain on resisted dorsiflexion of the wrist. Note that with tennis elbow the joint looks normal and there is no loss of movement. Although injection is the therapy of choice (Fig. 109), if a patient refuses injection you can try an epicondylitis clasp, physiotherapy and ultrasound. A few patients not responding to injection therapy will require surgery.

With golfer's elbow the tender point is at the medial epicondyle, at the site of the common flexor insertion. The diagnosis can be confirmed by eliciting pain on resisted palmar flexion of the wrist. Be sure to identify the ulnar nerve (lying in a groove behind the medial epicondyle) before you inject, to ensure that you are well clear of its course.

Needle and preparation to use

Use a 25-gauge (25 G $\times \frac{5}{8}$ in orange) needle with 1–2 ml 1% lignocaine and 1 ml (40 mg) methylprednisolone.

Note: Some authors suggest using only hydrocortisone as the steroid for injection because of the problem of fat atrophy and depigmentation. However, the longer-acting depot steroids give better results and, provided they are injected deeply, rarely cause significant atrophy or depigmentation.

Injection technique

• Tennis elbow (Figs 110, 111). Before the injection warn the patient it might be painful and that the pain may persist for 24–48 hours. If the patient has an important event, or is driving a long distance, he may wish to postpone the treatment

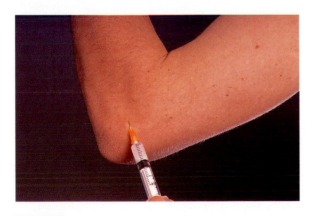

Fig. 109

Injection of a tennis elbow: one of the commonest sites for injection therapy.

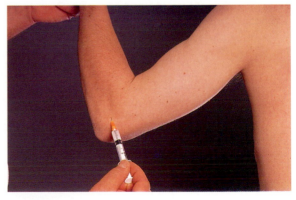

Fig. 110

Injecting a tennis elbow.

Injecting a tennis or golfer's elbow

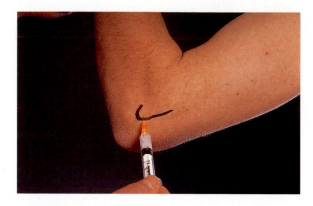

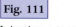

Injecting a tennis elbow.

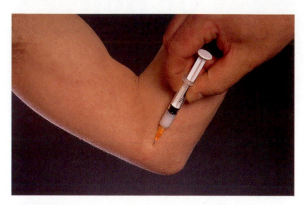

Fig. 112

Injecting a golfer's elbow.

until he has a relatively free day available following the injection.

First mark the tender area with your fingernail prior to swabbing. Inject the area of maximum tenderness. The injection is a subperiosteal one, under some pressure, injecting down to the bone. Once at the site inject small amounts several times, infiltrating over an area. It is more painful to inject as a single bolus.

• Golfer's elbow (Figs 112 and 113). Similar in principle to the above, but make sure to avoid the ulnar nerve!

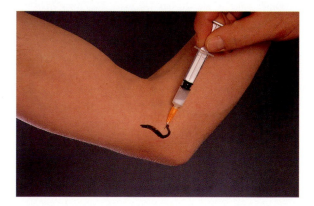

Fig. 113

Injecting a golfer's elbow.

23 Injecting a carpal tunnel syndrome

Injection for carpal tunnel syndrome is often combined with the use of a splint and diuretics. Surgery is recommended for those patients where injection fails to relieve the symptoms, or those with severe or chronic symptoms, including muscle wasting secondary to carpal tunnel syndrome.

Making the diagnosis

Carpal tunnel syndrome is caused by compression of the median nerve by the flexor retinaculum. It usually presents as pain associated with paraesthesiae in the distribution of the median nerve in one or both hands. The pain/paraesthesiae will be described in various ways, from a 'burning' pain to a 'pins and needles', and there can be some radiation of the pain to the forearm, or even as far as the shoulder. The symptoms are relieved by rest and worsened by use. The most characteristic feature is the worsening of the symptoms at night, causing the patient, usually a woman in middle age, to hang the arm out of bed to obtain relief. There may or may not be demonstrable numbness in the distribution of the median nerve. Muscle wasting of the thenar eminence is a sign only seen in advanced cases (where surgery rather than injection will be required).

The classic sign to confirm the diagnosis is Tinel's sign – reproducing the symptoms by tapping with a finger or tendon hammer over the site of the median nerve at the wrist. Reproducing the symptoms by pressing over the median nerve site while the patient palmar flexes is another confirmatory sign. If there is real doubt the response to injection can confirm the diagnosis – even electromyographic (EMG) testing cannot always provide the diagnosis prior to injection.

One must always remember that there are diseases associated with/causing carpal tunnel syndrome. The main ones to remember are hypothyroidism, a previous Colles fracture, rheumatoid arthritis, osteoarthritis of the wrist, psoriatic arthritis and fluid retention caused by drugs or pregnancy. Carpal tunnel syndrome can be associated with painful shoulder conditions, and there are associations with rarer conditions such as acromegaly and myelomatosis. Finally, remember to exclude a trapped nerve in the neck causing a painful hand with numbness of the middle finger, before injecting a supposed carpal tunnel syndrome.

Needle and preparation to use

Use a 25-gauge (25 G $\times \frac{5}{8}$ in orange) needle and 0.5–1 ml of methylprednisolone acetate (20–40 mg).

Note: Avoid local anaesthesia around the median nerve as this may itself produce numbness of the fingers.

Injection technique
(Figs 114, 115)

- Identify the surface landmarks, marking the position of the palmaris longus tendon and the median nerve (located immediately adjacent to and deep to the palmaris longus). With the patient's hand dorsiflexed, swab the area on the palmar surface of the hand to be injected and then insert the needle at a near horizontal angle

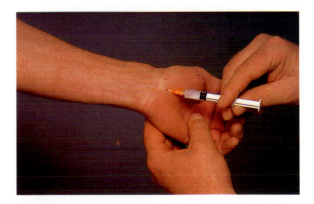

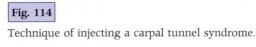

Technique of injecting a carpal tunnel syndrome.

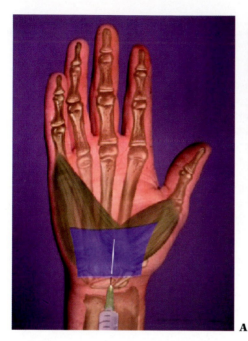

A

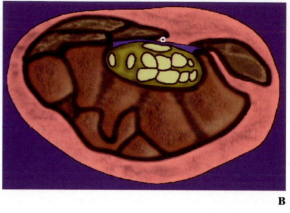

B

A Schematic representation of the carpal tunnel (shown in blue); **B** Cross-section of wrist.

about one-quarter of an inch to the ulnar side of the palmaris longus tendon (and clear of the median nerve) at the site of the wrist flexor palmar crease, marking where the hand joins the forearm.

- Advance the needle slowly through the flexor retinaculum until a loss of resistance is encountered and the steroid can be injected. Any resistance to injection means an incorrect siting of the needle and warrants repositioning of the injection. Similarly, if the patient experiences any

pain, numbness or paraesthesiae the median nerve may have been touched, so withdraw the needle slightly prior to injection. Note that if no palmaris longus tendon is present inject slightly to the ulnar side of the midpoint at the wrist flexor palmar crease. As with tennis elbow the injection may worsen symptoms for 24–72 hours initially. Relief is usually felt after a few days, improving progressively over the next 2 weeks. A wrist splint is useful for the first 2 weeks after the injection.

24 Injecting a trigger finger

There is little problem in diagnosing a trigger finger, the finger locking in flexion then unlocking with a characteristic click when it is forcibly extended. The thumb can also be affected (trigger thumb). The underlying pathology is a swelling of the flexor tendon which catches on the flexor sheath. This swelling can generally be felt on the palmar surface of the hand. Injecting steroid into the tendon sheath (*not* into the tendon, as this may cause tendon rupture) can be successful in curing the condition. Use a 25-gauge (25 G $\times \frac{5}{8}$ in orange) needle and 0.5 ml (20 mg) methylprednisolone acetate with 0.5 ml of 1% lignocaine.

Injection technique (Fig. 116)

• Palpate for the thickened area, usually just below the distal palmar crease. After swabbing insert the needle at an oblique angle distal to the trigger point and advance it proximally into the tendon sheath. There should be no resistance to injection (if there is the needle should be repositioned).

You can check whether the needle is in the tendon if it moves when the patient flexes his/her fingers. You can also ensure success by palpating the tendon sheath, which should swell as you inject. If the injection fails, an operation should be considered.

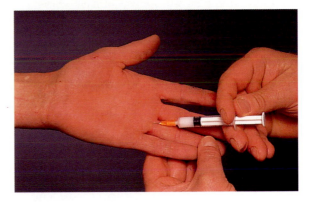

Fig. 116

Technique of injecting a trigger finger.

25 Injecting de Quervain's tenosynovitis

Making the diagnosis

With an increasing interest in work-related upper limb disorders such as tennis elbow, carpal tunnel syndrome and tenosynovitis, it is worthwhile acquiring a full range of injection skills for these disorders. De Quervain's tenosynovitis can arise from repetitive work and consists of pain, swelling and occasionally crepitus over the extensor pollicis longus (EPL) and abductor pollicis longus (APL) tendons (i.e. just proximal to the wrist on the radial side; see Fig. 117). The diagnosis is made by the history of the pain (including an occupational history or a history of injury) and the presence of localized tenderness, swelling or crepitus. Remember as always that the injection should be in the tendon sheaths not in the actual tendons. Also be sure you have located the nearby radial artery, and that your injection does not penetrate deeply to enter its wall. Use a 25-gauge (25 G $\times \frac{5}{8}$ in orange) needle and, 0.5–1 ml (20–40 mg) of methylprednisolone acetate plus 0.5–1 ml of 1% lignocaine.

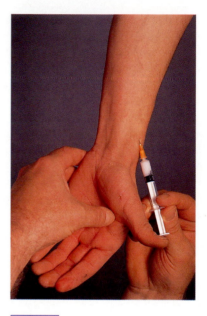

Fig. 117

Technique of injecting de Quervain's tenosynovitis.

Injection technique

First identify the EPL and APL tendons, the site of the crepitus and pain. After swabbing the area insert the needle just distal to the site, on the radial side of the wrist, advancing the needle obliquely and slowly into the synovial sheaths of the tendons (Fig. 117). Inject slowly – there should be no resistance to injection. If a resistance is felt you are likely to be hitting the tendon – withdraw slightly before injecting. You should be able to feel the tendon sheath swell as it is injected. If a large diffuse swelling appears over the site of injection, you are injecting subcutaneously and will need to try again. Injection usually affords immediate relief.

26 Injecting a plantar fasciitis

Plantar fasciitis is the commonest injection to be given in the foot. Note that Achilles tendinitis is not a simple injection because of the danger of tendon rupture, and it should not be attempted by the inexperienced.

Making the diagnosis

Plantar fasciitis is an inflammation of the insertion of the long plantar ligament into the calcaneum. It presents as a painful heel, with tenderness locally on palpation of the heel over the site of the ligament insertion. There may or may not be an associated calcaneal bony spur, and there is absolutely no need to X-ray – injection into the locally tender spot is all that is required. The spot to be injected should be marked beforehand and the patient should also be warned that the injection will be painful!

Plantar fasciitis can occur alone or in association with other conditions affecting joints, such as ankylosing spondylitis or Reiter's syndrome. Use a 21-gauge (21 G × 1½ in green) needle or a 23-gauge (23 G × 1 in blue) needle and 3 ml of 1% lignocaine plus 1 ml (40 mg) of methylprednisolone acetate.

Injection technique

Identify the tender spot. Use the lateral approach, as shown in Figure 118. Some use the plantar

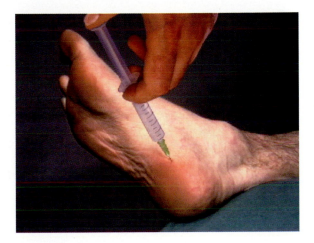

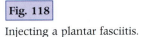

Injecting a plantar fasciitis.

approach but this is generally more painful. After swabbing the site, advance the needle from the side of the foot to the anterior border of the os calcis at the site of tenderness. Infiltrate widely around the ligament insertion.

27 Removing a foreign body from the eye

Whenever a patient presents with the possibility of a foreign body in the eye it is essential to take a proper history. Direct questions should be asked to exclude the history of a metallic foreign body – was the patient hammering, chiselling or grinding metal when he felt something enter his eye? High-velocity flying metal particles can penetrate the eye and be very difficult to detect (and may not be detected by examination with a light and ophthalmoscope). If there is any suggestion of the possibility of a metallic foreign body, the patient should be referred at once to the eye department/eye casualty. Most foreign bodies will be specks of dirt and dust, easily removable by the following technique:

1. Identify the foreign body clearly. A full examination of the eye is essential, including fluorescein staining (always remove the patient's contact lenses before this procedure as contact lenses take up the stain). As well as showing any corneal ulceration, fluorescein will often provide a clue to the presence of a subtarsal foreign body by demonstrating characteristic scratch lines over the cornea, where the foreign body has abraded the cornea on blinking.

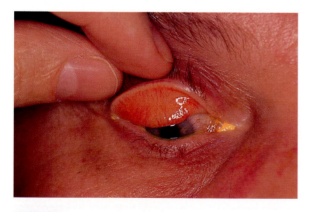

Fig. 119

Lid eversion: the patient must look downwards with both eyes open.

You should as a matter of routine check the vision, fundus and pupil, which should all be normal. Any abnormality detected raises the possibility of more serious eye trauma/disease, and merits referral.

2. The difficult part of the eye to gain acccess to is the portion under the upper lid. As this is a common site for a foreign body, the lid must always be everted. The technique of lid eversion is:
(i)   Ask the patient to look downwards as far as possible. During lid eversion they should continue to look down (Fig. 119).
(ii) Pull the eyelid outwards slightly, holding the eyelashes, then gently press a small glass rod down from above on the outside of the lid, everting the lid up and over the rod. All doctors should be familiar with this technique.

3. Foreign bodies revealed on lid eversion can usually be flicked off the lid with ease, using a cottonwool bud for example.

4. Removing a corneal foreign body may be a four-stage process:
(i)   First anaesthetize the eye with 0.5% amethocaine drops. Use the MINIMs disposable format (single dose) so as to avoid infection from previously opened bottles. The 'two drop' technique should be used. The first drop stings (warn the patient), resulting in lacrimation which washes out some of the drop; the second drop after 1 or 2 minutes will complete the anaesthesia.
(ii) After the cornea has been anaesthetized the foreign body can often be removed using a cottonwool bud (Fig. 120).
(iii) If the cottonwool bud does not succeed you will have to consider using a needle. Lay the patient flat (so they cannot fall forward accidentally) and, with a good light illuminating the foreign body, advance a green 21 G needle from the lateral side and, using the edge of the needle (never the tip), gently stroke the foreign body off the cornea (Fig. 121). **Do not use**

force; do not 'dig' into the cornea. If this is not easily achieved refer the patient to the eye clinic. It is far better to err on the side of being too gentle and admit defeat rather than dig into the cornea and cause trauma yourself.

(iv) After removal instill chloramphenicol ointment in the eye and pad the eye, removing the pad after 12 hours. If the patient would find a pad too uncomfortable, use chloramphenicol eye drops four times a day with the ointment at night for 2 days. This simple regimen assumes that you have been gentle with your removal efforts, inflicting no secondary damage. Patients should be told to report the following day if there is any pain, redness, discharge or visual disturbance. With a routine, gently performed removal this should not happen. If it does you will need to reassess, fluorescein stain and refer to the eye clinic.

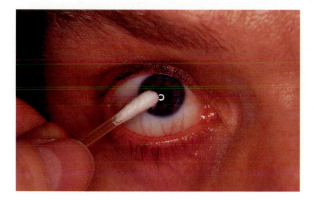

Fig. 120

Removing a foreign body with a cottonwool bud.

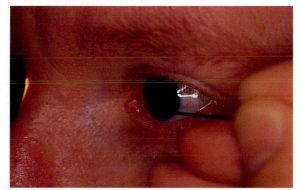

Fig. 121

Removing a foreign body by gentle stroking from the side with the edge of a green needle.

Removing a foreign body from the ear

The two most common scenarios here are an insect in the ear canal, and a child who has, with great dexterity, managed to insert some toy/household material into the ear canal.

The first task is to identify the nature of the foreign body. If it is an insect of some sort, kill it first by pipetting a few drops of alcohol into the ear canal.

Beware of vegetable matter (peas or mashed potato for instance!) before considering syringing, as these can take up water and swell, making removal even more difficult. Do *not* syringe vegetable matter: refer to hospital. If there is an obvious discrete inanimate foreign body, such as a small plastic toy, you may be able to remove it directly, pulling the pinna upwards and backwards to straighten the ear canal and using a hook passed along the floor of the external auditory meatus and behind the foreign body. By rotating the hook and using gentle traction the foreign body can be removed. Alternatively you may be able to remove

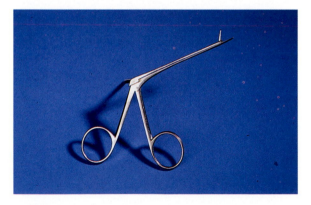

Fig. 122

Crocodile forceps.

it with special crocodile forceps (Fig. 122). Do not chase the foreign body down the ear canal: if you cannot remove it easily, desist and refer the patient to the ENT department. Similarly, if a foreign body lies adjacent to the tympanic membrane refer to the ENT department rather than risk perforating the drum.

For smaller, smoother, rounded objects lodged further down the ear canal, or dead insects, ear syringing is the more appropriate technique. The standard ear syringing technique is used, directing the jet of warm water upwards and backwards along the canal.

Finally, do not attempt to remove a foreign body from the ear of a child under the age of 3 – the risk of inflicting trauma is too great. Refer these children to hospital.

Removing a foreign body from the nose

The patient here is almost invariably a child who has inserted a foreign body up the nose. A unilateral nasal discharge in a child strongly points to the possibility of an intranasal foreign body. Before removing the foreign body, check the other nostril and the ears for further surprises!

A useful technique to remove foreign bodies from the nose is as follows:

1. Wrap the child tightly in a blanket and instruct the parent to hold him or her upright (Fig. 123).
2. An assistant holds the head while the examiner places a probe towards the roof of the nose to get above the foreign body, an auriscope illuminating the procedure.
3. At a given signal the assistant lets go of the child's head; the child will recoil his head backwards, thus allowing the examiner to flick the foreign body out of the nostril (Fig. 124).

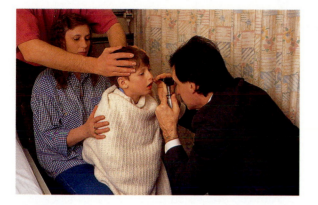
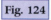

Fig. 123

Technique of removing a foreign body from the nose of a child.

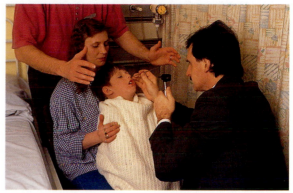

Fig. 124

Technique of removing a foreign body from the nose of a child.

Nasal cautery

The treatment of an acute epistaxis is to instruct the patient to lean forward, pinching the nostrils between finger and thumb continuously for 10 minutes while they breathe through the mouth. A sponge soaked in cold water or an ice pack over the bridge of the nose will help stem the blood flow. If this strategy fails, you may need to pack the nose or use a balloon device.

In younger patients the bleeding generally comes from a group of dilated blood vessels in Little's area, an area of the septum easily visualized with a speculum. More elderly patients may bleed from the posterior nasal passages, and the nose bleeds here can be associated with hypertension. Severe epistaxes in the elderly can be more difficult to control.

A relatively common scenario is a patient, usually a child, with recurrent epistaxes, and here the technique of nasal cautery is helpful. In any such patient it is, of course, sensible first to ensure that there is no bleeding diathesis. Nasal cautery should be an elective procedure in between bleeding episodes.

Technique

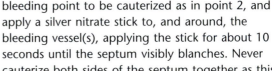

There is no particular age limit for nasal cautery, although children under 4 rarely sit still sufficiently long for proper treatment and are best referred to hospital if cautery is required.

1. Position the patient sitting upright, head tilted.

2. With your thumb on the tip of the patient's nose you should be able to upturn the nostril sufficiently to see the area to be cauterized, your nurse directing a light source to illuminate and identify the bleeding point. Alternatively, a nasal speculum can be used (Fig. 125).

3. Anaesthetize the area to be cauterized by using a pledget of cotton wool soaked in 2 ml of 10% topical cocaine solution and leaving it in contact with the septum to be cauterized for 10 minutes prior to cautery.

4. Remove the cottonwool pledget, reilluminate the bleeding point to be cauterized as in point 2, and apply a silver nitrate stick to, and around, the bleeding vessel(s), applying the stick for about 10 seconds until the septum visibly blanches. Never cauterize both sides of the septum together as this can cause perforation. Figure 126 shows an adequate cautery.

5. Warn the patient that for the next 24 hours there may be some blackish silver nitrate material or spots of blood running down the nostril.

6. Review at 6 weeks, by which time full healing should have occurred. If not you may try a further cautery – but if this fails to work the patient is best referred to hospital for electrocautery.

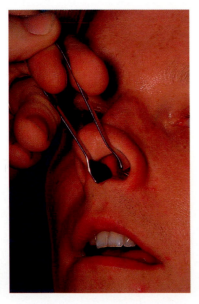

Fig. 125
Examining the nose with a speculum.

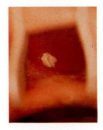

Fig. 126
The bleeding area of the nose adequately cauterized.

Aspiration of cysts and bursae

Aspiration of a cyst or bursa should be one of the procedures in the repertoire of every doctor offering minor surgery services. As always, the key to success is (1) to limit your endeavours to those cysts/bursae which can be reasonably dealt with without major risk of serious infection or damaging sequelae; (2) to be absolutely sure of your anatomy before proceeding; and (3) to use a scrupulous aseptic technique. A green 21 G × 1½ in needle is adequate for most aspirations.

Types of cyst/bursa suitable for aspiration as a safe minor surgical procedure include breast cysts, epididymal cysts, thyroid cysts, a spermatocoele, an olecranon bursa, prepatellar bursitis (housemaid's knee) and a semimembranosus bursa (Baker's cyst).

Breast cyst

Use a 20 ml syringe with a green needle. Stabilize the cyst between your fingers (Fig. 127), clean the skin with cetrimide or a swab at the site of the anticipated puncture, then insert the needle

through the skin into the cyst (Fig. 128). Aspirate the cyst (Fig. 129) until it can no longer be felt, and then withdraw the needle, pressing firmly on the exit point with a swab as the needle is removed. Palpate to ensure you have fully drained the cyst. If it is still palpable after aspiration refer for a

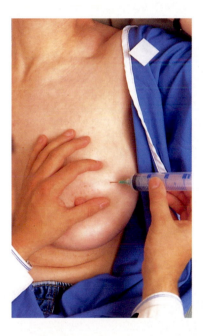

Fig. 128

Inserting the needle.

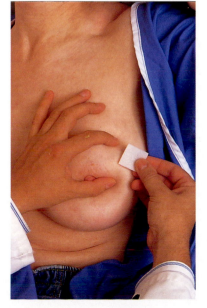

Fig. 127

Stabilizing a breast cyst between the fingers.

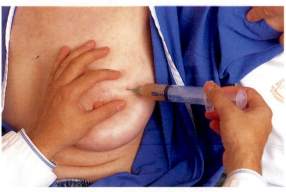

Fig. 129

Aspirating the cyst.

Aspiration of cysts and bursae

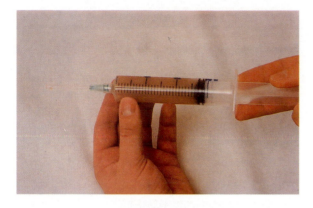

The typical yellow-brown fluid obtained from a breast cyst.

consultant opinion; if not, review the patient after 2–3 weeks. The fluid aspirated (Fig. 130), should be sent for cytology in a pot containing an alcohol-based fixative/preservative (as for fine needle aspirates – an 'FNA' histology pot). Bloodstaining of the fluid is a sign that the 'cyst' may not be benign. Note that there is no evidence that attempting to aspirate a cyst will spread a malignancy.

Epididymal cyst

Small epididymal cysts need not be aspirated as they rarely cause symptoms. If they are multiple they may need referral to a consultant surgeon. The technique is as for a breast cyst.

Thyroid cyst

A thyroid cyst can be aspirated in the same way as for breast cysts. Bleeding and haematoma formation are the commonest complications. The fluid should be sent for histology. Note that if you are at all

unsure about a thyroid swelling, ultrasound will be useful in determining the diagnosis.

Olecranon bursa

Small bursae may be left alone to resolve naturally. As with breast cysts, use a 20 ml syringe with a green needle, swab the skin with alcohol, pierce the skin with the needle, aspirate until flat and then withdraw the needle, applying pressure to the exit site. To prevent recurrence two strategies can be employed: (1) firm bandaging for at least 72 hours following aspiration, encouraging the patient to gently move the arm within this restraint – this is essential after all aspirations at this site; (2) if the bursa recurs after the simple procedure outlined above you can try injecting 20–40 mg of methylprednisolone into the site after aspiration, but *only* if the fluid withdrawn is a clear, straw yellow colour, i.e. there is no sign of infection.

Prepatellar bursitis

Exactly the same principles apply as with an olecranon bursa, including the need for firm bandaging after aspiration and the absolute rule to inject the 40 mg of methylprednisolone into the site *only* if the fluid withdrawn is clear, with no evidence of infection. Be particularly wary of introducing infection at this site.

Semimembranosus bursa (Baker's cyst (Fig. 131))

This is a site with important anatomy, not least the popliteal artery. Bleeding is a particular risk here. Aspiration (Figs 132, 133) follows the principles for aspiration of the other bursae, but even with these precautions recurrence is common and operative intervention may subsequently be required.

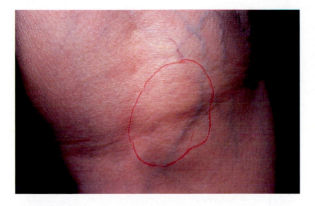

Fig. 131

Typical position of a semimembranosus bursa (Baker's cyst).

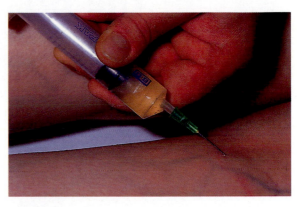

Fig. 132

Green needle and large syringe used to aspirate the contents of the cyst.

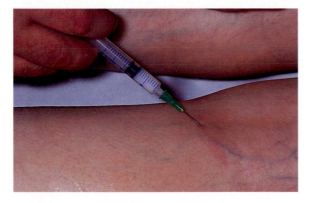

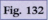

Fig. 133

After detaching the syringe (leaving the needle in the cyst) 2 ml of methylprednisolone are instilled.

31 Fine needle aspiration of the breast

This is another valuable technique for the family practitioner to master. In fact, fine needle aspiration can also be of value in thyroid lumps and lymph nodes.

The object of fine needle aspiration is to obtain a core of tissue for histological examination. There is little point in aspirating an obviously ulcerating breast carcinoma – these can be referred directly to hospital.

Since cytology is the aim, you must ensure that you have available special FNA histology pots containing a fixative/preservative which will fix and preserve cells during their transport to the laboratory.

Technique

1. Lay the patient down in a comfortable position.

2. Isolate the lesion (Fig. 134) between the thumb and finger of your non-dominant hand.

3. Clean the skin with cetrimide.

4. Using a 10 ml syringe with a green 21 G $\times$ $1\frac{1}{2}$ in needle, insert the needle through the swabbed skin into the lesion (Fig. 135).

5. Apply reasonable suction to the syringe once the needle is in the lesion (Fig. 136). Rotate the needle in the lesion and release the suction.

6. Withdraw slightly from the lesion but keep the needle in the breast tissue. Reinsert into the lesion and once again suck, rotate and release. Repeat this two or three times (the object being to obtain small cores of tissue within the lumen of the needle).

7. Withdraw the needle from the breast, covering the puncture site with an adhesive dressing.

8. Irrigate the syringe and needle with the fixative/preservative in the histology pot (Fig. 137) to ensure that all the tissue enters the pot. Before dispatching to the laboratory label the pot and provide details of the site and consistency of the lump, together with a brief history of the patient's symptoms.

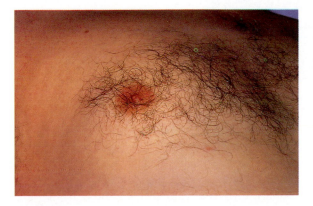

Fig. 134

A male breast with a subareolar mass.

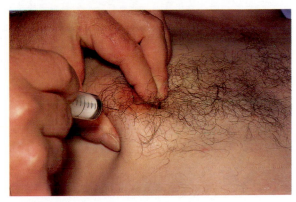

Fig. 135

Stabilizing the lump between thumb and forefinger and inserting the needle.

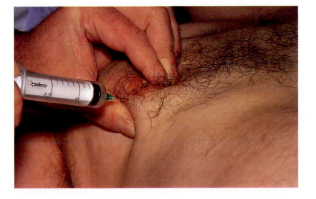

Fig. 136

Applying a vacuum to the needle, with a suction and rotation action as described in the text.

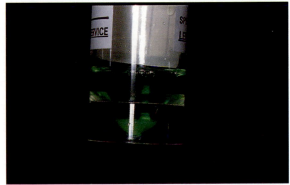

Fig. 137

The histology pot containing Cytospin fluid.

32 Draining a hydrocoele or spermatocoele

Hydrocoeles are common scrotal swellings and can grow to a large size. Many hydrocoeles, particularly in the elderly infirm, can be quite satisfactorily managed by aspiration. It is unwise to attempt treating hydrocoeles in children – these should be reserved for the specialist. The tapping of a hydrocoele is usually a recurrently performed procedure unless you use the phenolization technique described below. Hydrocoeles can be managed following a 10-point plan, as follows:

1. Make sure of your diagnosis. Before proceeding, ensure that you are dealing with a hydrocoele and not a hernia, cystic or solid tumour or varicocoele. The key points to ensure are (a) that the swelling transilluminates (use a powerful torch in a darkened room): if it does not, order an ultrasound prior to any attempt at draining; (b) that the swelling is discretely confined to the scrotum and that you can close your fingers above it; (c) that the swelling is cystic and not solid. It is worth checking the testes first, although this may not be possible until the hydrocoele is drained.

2. Use a 50 ml syringe with a green needle or, especially for larger lesions, an i.v. cannula. Our practice is to use an i.v. cannula to prevent damage to the testes by inadvertent trauma.

3. Swab the skin with cetrimide.

4. Introduce the cannula into the hydrocoele slowly, taking care that the needle point does not touch any surface blood vessels and steadying the scrotal contents with the other hand. The needle point should enter without resistance. Once in the hydrocoele, remove the needle and attach the syringe. This method facilitates repeated withdrawing of fluid without the risk of a moving needle traumatizing the tissues.

5. Withdraw the fluid, which should be clear and straw coloured. You may be withdrawing 100–200 ml of fluid, again emphasizing the usefulness of a cannula attached to a syringe (which can be emptied at intervals).

6. Aspirate until there is virtually no fluid left. At this stage, if you are using a green needle and not a cannula, there is a risk of piercing the testis, so take particular care.

7. Withdraw the cannula (or needle), applying pressure over the site of withdrawal with a swab. Palpate the scrotum and testis for any underlying abnormality. The patient should be instructed to wear tight underpants for support following the drainage procedure.

8. As a counsel of perfection the fluid aspirated would be sent off for cytology but, especially with a recurrent hydrocoele, one may feel confident in omitting cytology in routine cases, provided the aspirate is typically clear straw-coloured hydrocoele fluid.

9. The main danger is bleeding with the formation of a scrotal haematoma which, if large enough, may itself require subsequent drainage. Position the needle carefully to avoid unnecessary trauma.

10. You may be happy repeating this procedure every few months (or, of course, referring the patient subsequently for definitive surgery). A useful technique to avoid recurrence is to instill 10% phenol in water into the hydrocoele sac after aspiration before removing the needle. For an average-size hydrocoele about 5–10 ml of 10% phenol in water can be instilled.

Spermatocoeles can be treated identically (Figs 138–141), although volumes will be smaller and phenol is almost never required.

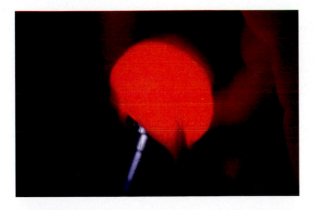

Fig. 138

A spermatocoele transilluminated.

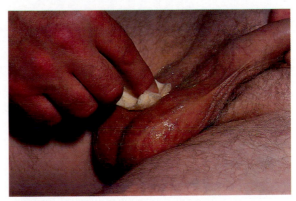

Fig. 139

Cleaning the scrotal skin with cetrimide.

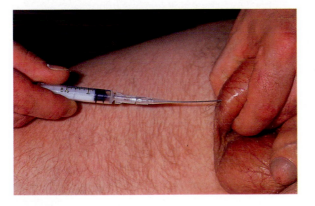

Fig. 140

Inserting the i.v. cannula into the spermatocoele.

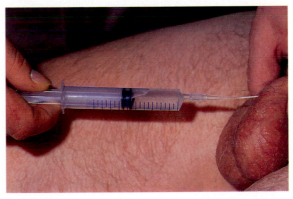

Fig. 141

The needle and small syringe have been replaced by a larger syringe to drain the spermatocoele.

33 Incising and draining abscesses

A common minor surgical procedure is the incision and draining of abscesses. Abscesses can occur at almost any site in the body. The following principles apply to their management:

1. First consider the cause of the abscess and its possible relation to underlying pathology. It is prudent to test the urine for diabetes in patients presenting with large, recurrent or unusual abscesses. The elderly in particular should be tested for glycosuria, as such an abscess is commonly the first presenting feature of diabetes. One might also have to consider the possibility of an immune deficiency, of whatever cause. Abscesses may be the marker of more widespread disease, for example the perianal abscesses associated with Crohn's disease.

2. Consider next the size and location of the abscess. Very large or deep abscesses may need to be drained under general anaesthetic. There are also sites where the abscess is best dealt with by a consultant surgeon because of difficult access or possible complications. Abscesses to refer to a consultant surgeon are those in the breast, ischiorectal abscesses, perianal abscesses, pilonidal abscesses and abscesses on the face.

3. As part of your assessment look for surrounding cellulitis. If there is a surrounding cellulitis the patient should be considered for referral to hospital for intensive antibiotic treatment prior to (or in addition to) any surgery. Cellulitis is a potentially dangerous condition, not to be underestimated.

4. If you are happy with draining the abscess the technique to follow is:
(i)   Spray the crown of the abscess with ethyl chloride spray (Fig. 142).
(ii) Incise the pointing tip of the abscess (Fig. 143).
(iii) Squeeze out the contents of the abscess, breaking down any loculi within it with a curette (Fig. 144).
(iv) Pack the cavity left (Fig. 145) with a paraffin gauze dressing.
(v)   Dress daily until healed.
Note that routine antibiotics are not usually required.

5. Note that paronychiae are not necessarily simple to incise – the infected abscess may spread under the nail and need proper drainage. Similarly, pulp abscesses can extend deeply and require a more formal surgical approach.

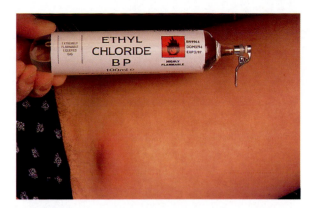

Fig. 142

Ethyl chloride is sprayed over the crown of the abscess to effect anaesthesia.

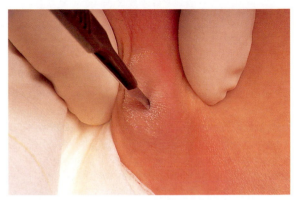

Fig. 143

A cruciate incision is made over the pointing tip of the abscess.

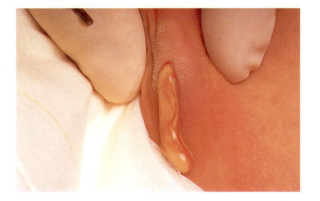

Fig. 144

Free drainage of pus from the abscess.

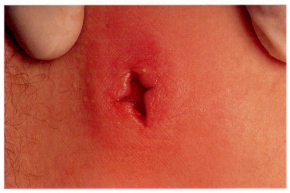

Fig. 145

A clean abscess cavity to be packed, e.g. with a paraffin gauze dressing.

34 Biopsy of skin lesions

Skin biopsy is a minor surgery technique that is occasionally useful in specific situations, for example in determining the diagnosis of a large lesion (e.g. a patch of (?) Bowen's disease on the leg) before deciding on treatment. Skin biopsy should, however, be used with discretion: if you see a patient with a pigmented lesion that has any possibility of being a malignant melanoma, you should refer the patient urgently to a dermatologist rather than trying to biopsy the lesion.

There are three forms of skin biopsy.

1. **Excision biopsy** (Figs 146–49). As the name implies, this means excising the whole lesion and sending it for histology. Excision biopsy is suitable for small lesions (i.e. less than about 1 cm in diameter) which are not placed over tight areas of

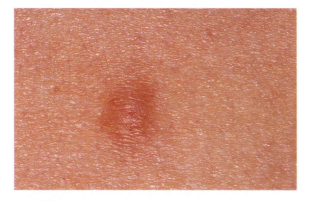

Fig. 146

A (?) histiocytoma of the leg. Excision required for confirmation of the diagnosis.

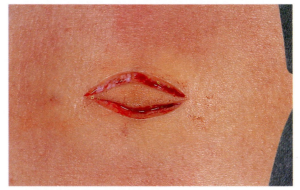

Fig. 147

An elliptical incision is made allowing for a good margin of normal skin around the lesion.

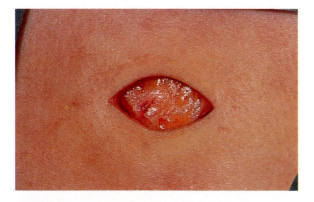

Fig. 148

The specimen has been removed with forceps, orientated and put into a formalin pot (see text).

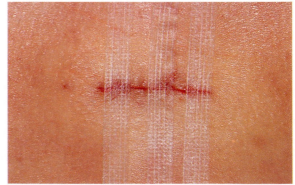

Fig. 149

Closure with subcorticular Vicryl and skin closure strips.

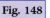
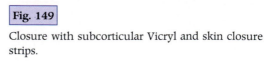

skin (e.g. the nose, the ears). Lesions on the face are best left to the specialist.

The technique of excision biopsy is:

(i) After skin cleansing with cetrimide infiltrate 1% lignocaine into the ellipse of skin where the incision will be made. Do not infiltrate the lesion directly as this will disrupt the histology.

(ii) Make an elliptical incision along Langer's lines, allowing a margin of 3 mm of normal skin around the lesion. It is essential to excise the lesion completely, with a margin of normal skin around it.

(iii) To orientate the specimen for the histopathologist mark one edge, e.g. the left lateral edge, with a skin stitch.

(iv) Incise down to fat, so that in excising the lesion you have gone deep enough to remove the whole lesion together with some underlying fatty tissue.

(v) After dissecting the lesion free put the whole lesion (still containing the orientating stitch) into a formalin pot and send it straight to the laboratory, together with full details of site, orientation, history and symptoms. The more you can tell the pathologist the easier it will be for him or her to report. Note that it is essential to obtain a full-thickness section for analysis.

(vi) One or two simple stitches with a monofilament suture should be all that is required to close the gap in the skin. For larger lesions that have been removed you may need to approximate the skin edges first with subcuticular undyed Vicryl.

2. **Incision biopsy.** For larger lesions an incision biopsy may be carried out. You must choose a typical area of the lesion, excise down to the fatty tissue underneath (as above), and extend the incision to include an area of normal skin for comparison. The technique of punch biopsy is easier and preferred by many to incision biopsy.

3. **Punch biopsy.** An easily carried out, effective way of obtaining a skin biopsy from a large lesion or rash. The technique is as follows:

(i) Choose a representative area of the rash/lesion (Fig. 150). You will be taking a biopsy of the lesion only, not lesion plus normal skin.

(ii) Using aseptic technique clean the area with cetrimide then anaesthetize superficially where the punch biopsy will enter, with 1% lignocaine plus adrenaline. Adrenaline must, of course, never be used on the extremities (fingers, toes, nose, ears, penis).

(iii) When anaesthesia is sufficient hold the biopsy punch (Fig. 151) vertical to the skin and, using a gentle twist, push the punch into the skin until you reach the depth needed to penetrate the underlying fatty tissue.

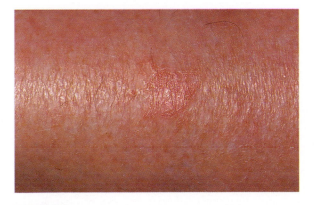

Fig. 150

An unusual scaly area on the leg. (?) diagnosis.

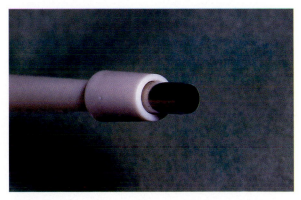

Fig. 151

The biopsy punch.

Biopsy of skin lesions

(iv) Remove the punch, leaving a core of tissue in the skin (Fig. 152). This can then be gently freed with a skin hook, cutting through the fatty base with scissors, and lifted clear of the skin (Fig. 153).

(v) The skin biopsy is sent for analysis as above, in a formalin histology pot, together with full details of site, symptoms, lesion's appearance etc.

(vi) The disc-shaped wound remaining after biopsy can be closed with a monofilament suture (e.g. Prolene). Remove the sutures in 5–7 days' time.

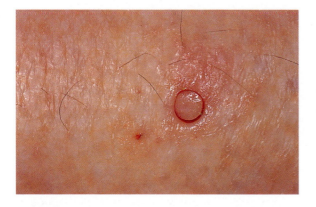

Fig. 152

The biopsy punch removed, leaving a core of tissue in the skin.

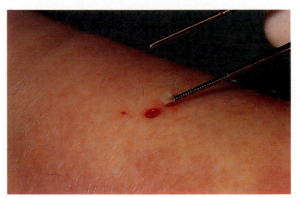

Fig. 153

The biopsy being lifted clear of the skin with forceps. The skin is then closed with a monofilament suture.

Inserting an oestrogen implant

Oestradiol implants are one option for hormone replacement therapy. Note that although they are used alone in hysterectomized women, women with an intact uterus will need to take monthly oral progestogen (e.g. norethisterone 5 mg twice daily for 10 days from the 15th day of each month) to achieve a withdrawal bleed, thus preventing endometrial hyperplasia. We do not use the implants for women with a uterus, not least because compliance with the progestogen tablets may present a problem, leaving the woman incorrectly receiving unopposed oestrogen. The main advantage of oestrogen implants is that there is no need for daily pills or patches. The main disadvantages are the need for progestogen in women with a uterus, the difficulties in discontinuing the preparation, and tachyphylaxis – a tendency for symptoms to return earlier and earlier between implants.

In the UK oestradiol implants come in three sizes: 25 mg, 50 mg and 100 mg. We use 100 mg inserted 3–6-monthly, the patient booking their own appointment for insertion according to symptoms. The implant is inserted subcutaneously in the anterior abdominal wall at the bikini line right, left or centre in position.

Technique of insertion

1. Cleanse the skin with cetrimide.
2. Infiltrate the area of insertion with 2–3 ml of 1% lignocaine, infiltrating deeply to the skin, subcutaneously along the line where you will be introducing the trocar.
3. With a size 15 blade make a small (about 7.5 mm) cut along Langer's lines in the skin, down to fat.
4. Open up the incision by inserting Mosquito forceps (Fig. 154) and using them to open up a channel for the trocar (Fig. 155) to pass.
5. Position the trocar and cannula in the subcutaneous space you have fashioned (Fig. 156).

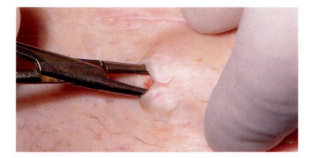

Fig. 154

Opening up the incision made using mosquito forceps.

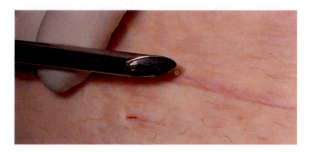

Fig. 155

Tip of the trocar and cannula.

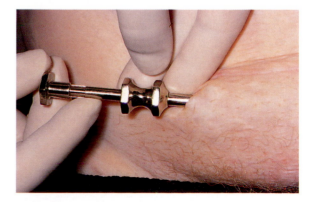

Fig. 156

Trocar and cannula inserted into the incision, prior to removing the trocar.

6. Remove the trocar, leaving the cannula in the space. Drop the oestrogen pellet (or pellets, if using the 75 mg dose) down the cannula. Use the obturator to ensure that the pellets fully traverse the cannula to arrive at their destination in the subcutaneous space.
7. Remove the cannula, applying firm pressure over the exit site. This leaves the pellet(s) in their subcutaneous pocket and a tiny surface wound.
8. The small surface wound can be closed with a single monofilament suture (Fig. 157).

Complications

1. Bleeding as a result of careless technique or too deep an incision.
2. Egression of the pellet, which may appear in the wound if the pocket is too shallow.
3. The pellets may form nodular lumps under the skin, necessitating their removal.

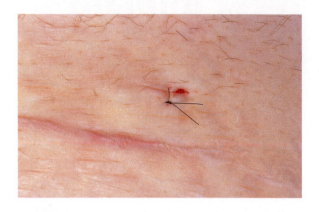

Fig. 157

Closure with 4/0 Prolene.

36 Vasectomy

The surgical technique of vasectomy should be well within the capacity of a family doctor. It is important to ensure that the patient and his partner are properly counselled before the operation, and it is helpful to design your own counselling checklist, as shown below.

The patient and his partner should be warned that (a) vasectomy is an irreversible procedure (it is difficult to successfully reverse a vasectomy: even in the best centres there is only a 50% chance of reversal within 2 years of the operation) and (b) there is a remote possibility of failure (due to recanalization or reduplication of the vas). Note from the checklist that the partner should be asked if she is awaiting a gynaecological operation – if she is already due for a laparoscopy it might be sensible for her to be sterilized at the same time rather than proceed with vasectomy. It is worthwhile asking the patient if he has fainted at any previous surgical procedures: vasovagal attacks may occur as a result of operating at this site, and if a patient is prone to

fainting he is best referred for operation in a hospital setting.

Written consent must be obtained, ideally from both partners, confirming that the patient has received and understood the information given in counselling. There is no absolute requirement for both parties to consent to vasectomy, but it is sensible and our practice to obtain consent from both. Sample wording of a consent form is shown in Figure 170. An instruction leaflet should be given to each patient undergoing vasectomy (Fig. 171).

Technique of vasectomy

This is demonstrated in Figures 158–169. There are several points worth emphasizing:

1. Ensure that you are adequately trained by a competent surgeon before setting out on your own. Vasectomy has an avoidable complication rate and success depends on good surgical technique.

```
Vasectomy counselling checklist

Name and age . . . . . . . . . . . . . . . . . . . . . . . . . . . . . . . . . . . . . . . . . . . . . . .
Telephone number . . . . . . . . . . . . . . . . . . . . . . . . . . . . . . . . . . . . . . . . . . .
Wife's name and age . . . . . . . . . . . . . . . . . . . . . . . . . . . . . . . . . . . . . . . . . .
Age and sex of children . . . . . . . . . . . . . . . . . . . . . . . . . . . . . . . . . . . . . . .
. . . . . . . . . . . . . . . . . . . . . . . . . . . . . . . . . . . . . . . . . . . . . . . . . . . . . . . . . .
Wife ? pregnant . . . . . . . . . . . . . . . . . . . . . . . . . . . . . . . . . . . . . . . . . . . . .
Expected delivery date . . . . . . . . . . . . . . . . . . . . . . . . . . . . . . . . . . . . . . .
Wife ? awaiting a gynaecological operation . . . . . . . . . . . . . . . . . . . . . .
Previous operations . . . . . . . . . . . . . . . . . . . . . . . . . . . . . . . . . . . . . . . . .
Drugs and allergies . . . . . . . . . . . . . . . . . . . . . . . . . . . . . . . . . . . . . . . . .
Past medical history of mumps/orchitis . . . . . . . . . . . . . . . . . . . . . . . . .
Date of operation . . . . . . . . . . . . . . . . . . . . . . . . . . . . . . . . . . . . . . . . . . .
Details of operation . . . . . . . . . . . . . . . . . . . . . . . . . . . . . . . . . . . . . . . . .
Specimens sent . . . . . . . . . . . . . . . . . . . . . . . . . . . . . . . . . . . . . . . . . . . .
Letter to doctor . . . . . . . . . . . . . . . . . . . . . . . . . . . . . . . . . . . . . . . . . . . .
```

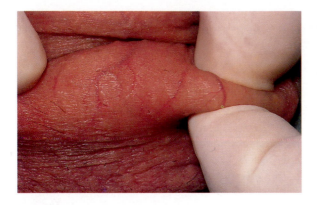

Fig. 158

The vas is identified and grasped between the fingers.

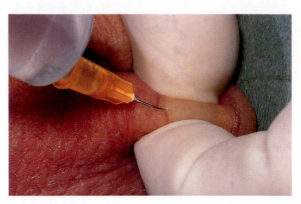

Fig. 159

Vas and scrotal skin infiltrated with 1% lignocaine anaesthetic.

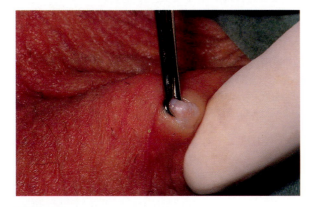

Fig. 160

Incision made over, and exposing, the vas.

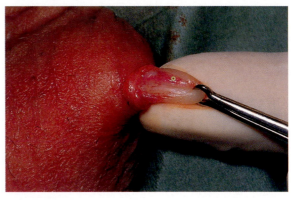

Fig. 161

The vas held in vasectomy forceps.

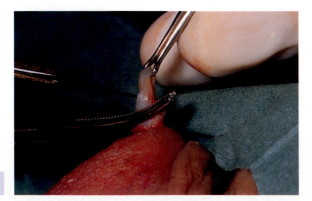

Fig. 162

After gentle dissection of superficial vessels, separating them from the vas, clips are applied to the proximal and distal ends of the vas prior to cautery.

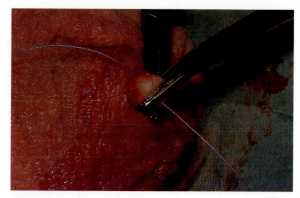

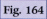

Fig. 163

Close-up showing typical end of vas.

Fig. 164

The distal end of the vas is now turned over and tied back on itself with Vicryl.

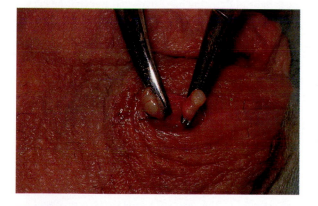

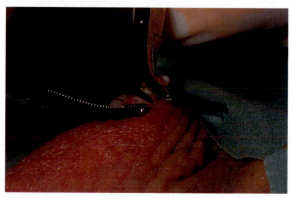

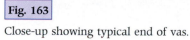

Fig. 165

Proximal and distal ends of vas prior to cautery.

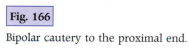

Fig. 166

Bipolar cautery to the proximal end.

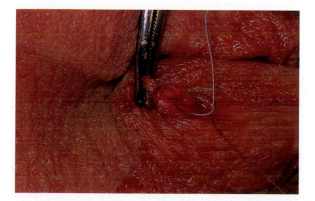

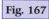

Fig. 167

After cautery the proximal end is allowed to slide back into the sheath and the sheath is closed with Vicryl.

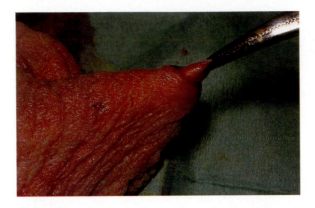

Fig. 168

With the divided vas allowed to sink back into the scrotum, the dartos muscle is grasped with a pair of forceps prior to wound closure.

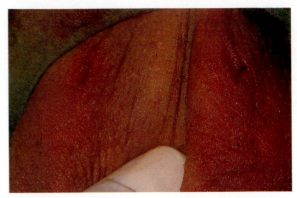

Fig. 169

The symmetrical bilateral scrotal wounds following stitching of the dartos muscle on each side following vasectomy. After vasectomy patients are advised to wear tight underpants for 2 days and to avoid heavy lifting for 2–3 days.

2. If the patient has not shaved off his pubic hair beforehand, it is wise to do so immediately before the operation.

3. Place adequate draping around the site, leaving only the scrotum visible to the operating surgeon.

4. Before you start operating palpate the testes and vas to finally exclude any pathology (although this should have been already completed before this stage). Beware the patient with a varicocoele!

5. Clean the scrotum and surrounding area thoroughly with cetrimide before injecting local anaesthetic.

6. When injecting local anaesthetic and handling the scrotum be gentle and inject the lignocaine slowly – this is the commonest part of the procedure to generate a faint, bradycardia or even a tonic–clonic seizure.

7. Since there is a definite risk of fainting, bradycardia or a fit, never perform a vasectomy unless you have an assistant present and an emergency resuscitation kit readily available.

8. Use absorbable sutures, e.g. Vicryl, throughout. Do not use non-absorbable sutures because of the risk of spermatic fistulae.

9. It seems pointless (unless the appearance is unusual) to send the removed vas for histology – assuming, of course, that you are sure it is the vas you have removed.

Postoperative care

The major complication is bleeding. A scrotal haematoma is a serious complication and can impair the viability of the testes (as well as causing the patient distress). Scrotal haematomas should be drained urgently, and this means having a colleague available out of hours who is capable of dealing with such a complication if the need arises. Note that this is a hospital procedure, invariably requiring a general anaesthetic, and should not be carried out in family practice. To reduce the risk of bleeding take meticulous care with haemostasis, clipping, ligating and cauterizing vessels as you go at the first sign of bleeding.

Wound infection is relatively rare with vasectomy, assuming you have used the sterile technique described. It usually responds to a course of antibiotics.

Following the operation arrangements have to be made for collection of semen samples. The patient

VASECTOMY

CONSENT BY A PATIENT TO OPERATION FOR PRIMARY STERILISATION

I (FULL NAME) . . . .

(ADDRESS) . . . .

. . . .

Consent to undergo the operation of vasectomy, the nature and effect of which have been explained to me by Dr. Cracknell. I have been told that the object of the operation is to make me sterile and incapable of fathering another child. I understand that two consecutive negative sperm counts must be obtained before I abandon other methods of contraception. I understand that there is a small risk of spontaneous reversal.

I consent to the administration of a local anaesthetic.

Signed . . . . Date . . . .

I confirm that I have explained to the patient and his wife/partner, the nature and effect of the operation and know of no contra-indications.

Signed . . . . Date . . . .

I . . . . of the above address, the wife/partner of . . . . hereby agree to the operation of vasectomy being carried out on my husband/partner, the nature and effect of which have been explained to me by Dr. Cracknell.

I have read and understood the whole of this form and it has been signed by my husband/partner in my presence.

Signed . . . . Date . . . .

Fig. 170

Vasectomy consent form.

Vasectomy

INSTRUCTIONS FOR PATIENTS UNDERGOING VASECTOMY

1. The day prior to your operation you should have a bath or a shower and shave off all of the pubic hair, this significantly reduces the risk of infection.

2. Kindly bring with you a tight pair of underpants, as compression reduces the incidence of bruising.

3. Immediately after your operation, whilst the anaesthetic is still effective, you will notice no discomfort. However, as the anaesthetic wears off you are likely to notice an aching sensation but this is usually all. Intense pain is uncommon and should be reported to me.

4. The operation of vasectomy is a minor procedure but even so it is unwise to drive before 24 hours or so after it is carried out.

5. A small amount of bruising and discharge from the wound is normal. Any significant bruising or discharge or swelling should be reported and either myself or one of my partners will see you.

6. Hundreds of millions of sperm are stored in the vas and seminal vesicle and are released over a period of weeks following your operation. It is therefore imperative that you continue with contraceptive measures until such time as two consecutive sperm counts have demonstrated no sperm and you have received a letter informing you that you are sterile.

7. Immediately after your operation, Sister will provide you with two pots and some instructions with them of how to take the samples and where to bring them. If there are difficulties attending on the due date, I would be most grateful if you could get in touch so that the date of your appointment may be altered.

8. If there is anything which causes concern, consequent upon this operation, please do not hesitate to get in touch. The number is . . . .

Fig. 171

Instructions for patients undergoing vasectomy.

should be supplied with two specimen pots for sperm counts at 8 and 12 weeks after the vasectomy, together with an instruction sheet for collecting the counts. It is vital that the patient understands how to collect the semen. The instruction sheet for collecting semen specimens for sperm counts should be similar to the example shown below.

Once the sperm counts are negative the patient should be sent a letter informing him of these results, as should the referring doctor if the patient is not generally under your care.

Instruction sheet for collecting seminal specimens for sperm counts

It is advisable to observe a 3-day period of abstinence before collecting the specimen.

Specimens may be collected by masturbation or by coitus interruptus (the withdrawal method).

The specimen container should be warmed to approximately body temperature before ejaculation, and maintained at that temperature for at least 15 minutes afterwards.

Allow the specimen to cool gradually and bring to the surgery within 2 hours of collection, between 5.30 and 6.30 pm on . . . .

NB: A specimen collected in a sheath is totally unsatisfactory.

---

37 Hyfrecating thread veins

A hyfrecator is only suitable for treating fine thread veins and is not suitable for venous lakes or varicose veins. It is used purely to obtain a good cosmetic result.

Technique (Figs 172–175)

Identify the thread veins and clean with cetrimide. Once dry, use a fine sharp hyfrecator needle to puncture the vein and then apply 0.2–0.4 W of power for about a second. Repeat this process along the thread veins at intervals. You may need 20–30 hyfrecations for a clutch of thread veins.

Postoperatively spray with Opsite. Warn the patient that there may be some scabbing over the veins as a result of the hyfrecations.

Review in 2–4 weeks to check the cosmetic result.

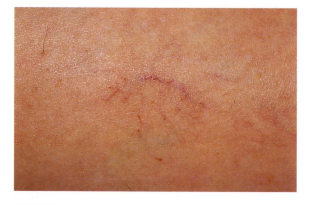

Fig. 172

Typical thread veins.

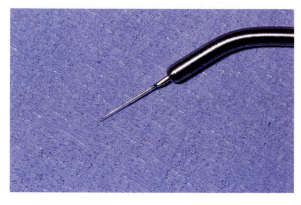

Fig. 173

A fine sharp hyfrecator needle.

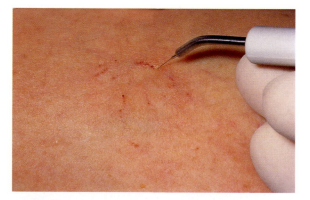

Fig. 174

The needle puncturing the vein at intervals, with 0.2–0.4 W of power applied for 1 second.

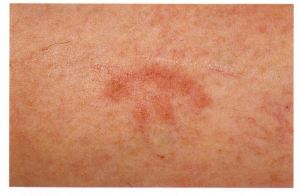

Fig. 175

Appearance immediately after treatment.

78

38 Dividing a penile frenulum

This is another example of a simple technique for a specific indication for minor surgery. The patient complained of splitting of the frenulum on intercourse, with pain and occasionally bleeding. The division of the frenulum relieved the symptoms. Note *never* to use adrenaline when operating at this site.

The technique is illustrated in Figures 176–179. Following the operation the patient should be advised to refrain from intercourse for 2–3 weeks, and to report back if there is any significant pain or bleeding.

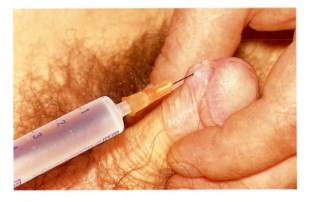

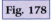
Fig. 176

Infiltration of 1–2 ml of 1% lignocaine into the frenulum.

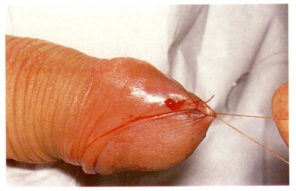

Fig. 177

Catgut sutures inserted on either side of the intended site of division.

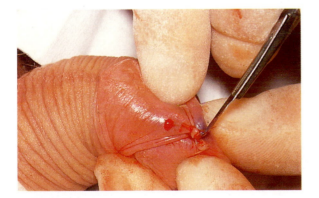

Fig. 178

Division between the catgut sutures with a size 15 blade.

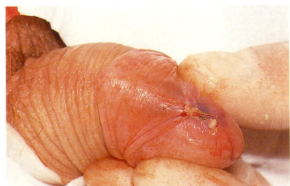

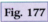
Fig. 179

Resulting divided frenulum between the sutures.

39 Haemorrhoids and their management

Haemorrhoids (piles) can present in various ways, including rectal bleeding, perianal pain, pruritus ani and as a perianal lump. They are basically engorged venous pads and the differential diagnosis will include a rectal or anal polyp, a skin tag and a rectal prolapse. Fissures, abscesses and fistulae are readily identifiable and should not pose a diagnostic problem.

Haemorrhoids can be classified as:

- First degree if they are restricted to the lower rectum and upper anal canal. These commonly cause the patient to present with rectal bleeding.
- Second degree if they prolapse after defaecation but are otherwise internally located.
- Third degree if they are prolapsed externally, independent of defaecation.

Patients presenting with rectal bleeding

All patients presenting with rectal bleeding must be adequately assessed to exclude a carcinoma/polyp. As a counsel of perfection this means a sigmoidoscopy in every case, but if there is an obvious bleeding haemorrhoid/anal tear in a low-risk patient, the lesion can be treated after rectal examination and proctoscopy, arranging follow-up after treatment. Sigmoidoscopy and perhaps a colonoscopy/barium enema will be essential in patients presenting with rectal bleeding who:

- are over 40 years of age
- have a change in bowel habit
- have blood mixed with mucus
- have associated abdominal pain
- have dark blood mixed with the stool rather than fresh red blood
- have a family history of polyps
- have substantial bleeding
- have recurrent or persistent bleeding
- have no identifiable external cause for their bleeding.

Management of haemorrhoids

Injection, banding or haemorrhoidectomy are all options, but many small haemorrhoids can be managed conservatively with a high-fibre diet (plus lactulose initially if the stools are hard) and a prescription for a topical steroid/local anaesthetic. Beware of sensitivity reactions to topical preparations, which can exacerbate pruritis.

Large prolapsing third-degree haemorrhoids may need surgical excision (haemorrhoidectomy) in hospital, but most other haemorrhoids of medium size or not responding to conservative measures can be dealt with in family practice. Thrombosed external piles (perianal haematomas) are common presentations and often resolve without surgical intervention. For a large acutely painful perianal haematoma a simple evacuation procedure will suffice.

Technique for draining a perianal haematoma

1. Position the patient in the left lateral position.
2. If local anaesthesia is required 2ml of 1% lignocaine can be used to infiltrate around the lesion. Ethyl chloride spray can be used as an alternative.
3. Incise the perianal haematoma with a number 10 blade.
4. Irrigate with normal saline.
5. Dress with a paraffin gauze dressing, covering this with an absorbent pack. Dress daily for a few days, ensuring that the patient bathes and cleans scrupulously after defaecation.

Injection of haemorrhoids

This is a useful technique to learn in family practice. You will require:

- A proctoscope with a good light source
- A haemorrhoid injection syringe with needle

- Oily phenol injection 5 ml ampoules × 2 (the BP preparation contains 5% phenol in a fixed oil).

Note that you will not require local anaesthesia.

Technique

- First position the patient in the left lateral position.
- Drape the patient to cover all but the anorectal region.
- Insert a gloved finger to check once more that there is no obvious rectal or anal pathology other than haemorrhoids.
- After withdrawing your finger, lubricate the proctoscope with KY jelly and insert gently to its full length.
- Withdraw the obturator from the proctoscope and illuminate. As the proctoscope is slowly and slightly withdrawn the haemorrhoids should be seen at the 3, 7 and 11 o'clock positions (Fig. 180A).
- Clearly identify the haemorrhoid you wish to inject. Inject above the dentate line (below is too painful), slowly and gently injecting 2–3 ml of oily phenol injection submucosally into the base of the pile (Fig. 180B). You should see the mucosa swell slightly as you inject. The patient feels no pain unless the injection is either too lowly placed or carried out too quickly. Occasionally a bleed will occur while injecting, but this is rarely of any

significance. Any oil spilt should be mopped up immediately. Complications should be few but include failure to achieve the required result, bleeding (if heavy this will need packing) and ulceration. Try not to inject the prostate gland! The procedure can be repeated at all three sites, giving a total volume of 10 ml (the maximum recommended in the British National Formulary for injection at any one time). The patient should be reviewed at 6 weeks, by which time the rectal bleeding should have resolved.

Banding of haemorrhoids
(Fig. 181)

Again a fairly simple technique, giving a rapid result without the use of any hazardous chemicals. Many prefer this technique to injection.
   You will require:

- A proctoscope with a good light source
- A Baron's banding device/applicator
- Rubber bands (Baron's bands)
- A pair of angled seizing forceps.

Technique

- Load the banding device with a rubber band.
- Position the patient in the left lateral position.
- Drape the patient to cover all but the anorectal region.

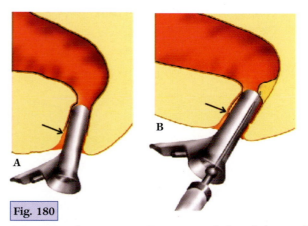

Fig. 180

A Insertion of proctoscope; B Injection of phenol above dentate line. Dentate line is shown by narrowing.

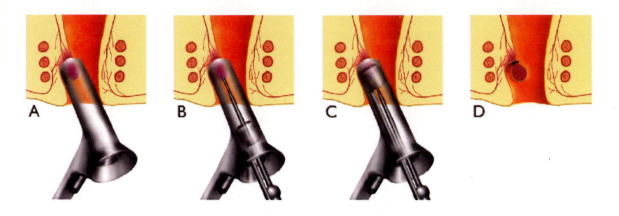

Fig. 181

A Haemorrhoid identified at tip of proctoscope; **B** Haemorrhoid grasped through bander; **C** Haemorrhoid pulled through bander prior to release of rubber band; **D** The banded haemorrhoid.

- Lubricate the proctoscope and insert to its full length.
- Remove the obturator and illuminate to demonstrate the haemorrhoids.
- Pass the banding device through the proctoscope.
- Pass the seizing forceps through the hole in the banding device.
- Identify the haemorrhoid to be banded and grasp it with seizing forceps above the dentate line (otherwise the procedure will be too painful).
- Using the forceps, pull the pile through the hole in the banding device. Make sure the neck of the pile is well into the banding device before releasing the rubber band. A particularly large pile may need two bands.
- Repeat the process with the other piles. After the procedure allow the patient to rest for a few minutes.

The major complications are pain, discharge and bleeding. A patient may experience quite considerable discomfort for up to about 48 hours after banding. Substantial haemorrhage is a rare but important complication.

The pile usually sloughs off in a few days – warn the patient that there will be some associated bleeding and discharge, which may last up to 10–14 days. Advise using a cottonwool pad or sanitary towel to protect clothing. You can review the patient in a week.

40 Sigmoidoscopy

This is a valuable technique for the family practitioner to master. In addition to patients presenting with rectal bleeding, the sigmoidoscope is of use in patients presenting with alterations in bowel habits (including unexplained diarrhoea or suspected colitis), in the follow-up of previously diagnosed and treated lesions (especially tubulovillous adenomas), and in the follow-up of patients with proctitis and ulcerative colitis.

Screening using sigmoidoscopy

The major use of sigmoidoscopy in the future may be for screening the population for colorectal cancer by once-only sigmoidoscopy at age 55–60, with colonoscopic surveillance for the 3–5% found to have high-risk adenomas. This screening regimen would prevent about 5500 colorectal cancers each year in the UK and 3500 deaths*. In the USA annual faecal occult blood testing with a sigmoidoscopy every 3–5 years is recommended from the age of 50 (Atkin et al 1993). The 65 cm flexible sigmoidoscope is recommended for screening, passing to the rectosigmoid junction and within reach of 60% of all colorectal cancers.

Types of sigmoidoscope

There are three types to consider:

1. The rigid sigmoidoscope. This is cheap, easy to use, and will last a lifetime in practice. Unfortunately it has a limited range, usually only passing to 15–20 cm. It is thus effectively only a rectoscope and will miss tumours higher up the sigmoid colon. If you are screening for colorectal cancer or have a patient in the higher-risk age group (say over 40), or have worrying features of rectal bleeding (e.g. dark blood mixed with the stool), a proper flexible

sigmoidoscope should be used. The rigid sigmoidoscope may have a place in the younger (e.g. under 40) patient, where fresh rectal bleeding is attributed to piles or (?) colitis and there is less risk of missing a carcinoma.

2. The plastic disposable sigmoidoscope. Ideal for family practice use but has exactly the same disadvantage as the rigid sigmoidoscope, i.e. a limited range.

3. The flexible fibreoptic sigmoidoscope. If there is any true likelihood of a colorectal cancer this is the sigmoidoscope of choice. It can pass up to 50–60 cm, within reach of 60% of all colorectal cancers. Unfortunately, it involves a heavy capital outlay (in terms of sterilization as well as cost).

Preparation for and technique of sigmoidoscopy (Figs 182–185)

No overnight preparation is required. About 30 minutes before the procedure the patient is given a phosphate enema.

1. Ensure that the sigmoidoscopy tray is set up. This should contain the sigmoidoscope, biopsy forceps, a formalin pot and KY jelly.

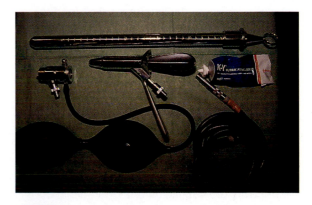

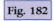

A tray prepared for sigmoidoscopy/proctoscopy.

---

* Atkin WS, Cuzick J, Northover JMA, Whynes DK Prevention of colorectal cancer by once-only sigmoidoscopy. Lancet 1993;341: 736–740.

Sigmoidoscopy

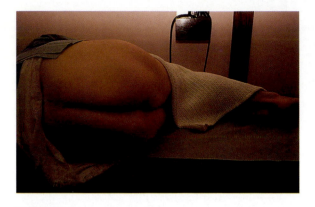

The patient in the left lateral position.

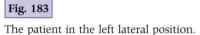

Fig. 184

Advancing the sigmoidoscope towards the umbilicus for about 3 cm.

2. Position the patient in the left lateral position.

3. Lubricate the end of the sigmoidoscope with KY jelly and insert gently into the anal canal, aiming for the umbilicus. Advance about 3–4 cm then move the sigmoidoscope so that the tip follows the curve of the sacrum. Remove the obturator and attach the light source. Using insufflated air, puff the mucosa away from the end of the sigmoidoscope to follow the lumen of the bowel. Some manoeuvring will be necessary to negotiate the folds of mucosa. Pass the sigmoidoscope, aiming to visualize as much bowel as possible. Negotiation of the rectosigmoid junction may be difficult and painful.

4. Any lesion found should be biopsied with the forceps, the level of the lesion recorded and the lesion sent for histology. A lesion should be biopsied more than once. Look at the stool above the sigmoidoscope to see if there is any evidence of bleeding coming from higher up: is the stool a normal colour or bloodstained? Look similarly at the mucosal appearance.

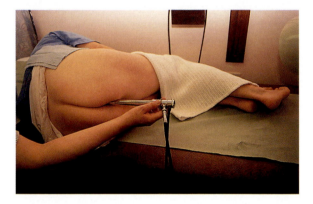

Fig. 185

Moving the sigmoidoscope so the tip follows the curve of the sacrum, under direct vision and insufflating with air as you go.

Complications of sigmoidoscopy include perforation of the bowel – avoided by gentle technique (never use force) – bleeding following biopsy and pain. The procedure is usually relatively painless. Occasionally the insufflation of air will mimic the symptoms of an irritable bowel syndrome.

If a sigmoidoscopy cannot adequately account for the patient's symptoms further investigation should be considered. If you are at all in doubt about your equipment or your ability to use a sigmoidoscope, refer the patient to hospital.

Index

Index